SUBSTANCE ABUSE ASSESSMENT, INTERVENTIONS AND TREATMENT

MARIJUANA: USES, EFFECTS AND THE LAW

SUBSTANCE ABUSE ASSESSMENT, INTERVENTIONS AND TREATMENT

Additional books in this series can be found on Nova's website under the Series tab.

Additional E-books in this series can be found on Nova's website under the E-books tab.

SUBSTANCE ABUSE ASSESSMENT, INTERVENTIONS AND TREATMENT

MARIJUANA: USES, EFFECTS AND THE LAW

ANDREA S. ROJAS
EDITOR

Nova Science Publishers, Inc.
New York

For permission to use material from this book please contact us:
Telephone 631-231-7269; Fax 631-231-8175
Web Site: http://www.novapublishers.com

LIBRARY OF CONGRESS CATALOGING-IN-PUBLICATION DATA

Marijuana : uses, effects and the law / [edited by] Andrea S. Rojas.
p. cm. -- (Substance abuse assessment, interventions and treatment)
Includes bibliographical references and index.
ISBN 978-1-61209-206-5 (hbk. : alk. paper)
1. Marijuana. 2. Marijuana abuse. I. Rojas, Andrea S.
HV5822.M3M35 2011
362.29'5--dc22
2010047016

Published by Nova Science Publishers, Inc. † New York

CONTENTS

PREFACE

The cannabis sativa plant, more commonly known as marijuana, has been used medicinally for millenia and continues to play a significant role in medical treatment today. This new book presents topical research in the study of marijuana; its uses, effects and legal issues. Topics discussed include measurement of cannabis consumption to assess the role of drug potency in rising rates of cannabis misuse disorders; the influence of marijuana legislation on vulnerable populations; marijuana use among adolescents and its effects and recreational marijuana use in a bariatric clinic population.

Chapter 1 - Rates of cannabis use are consistently reported as much higher in psychiatric samples than in the general population, with some studies reporting abuse rates as high as 42 % among people with schizophrenia. This association has led to several hypotheses: That cannabis may be a causal agent in the development of schizophrenia; that cannabis may trigger schizophrenia in people who are vulnerable to the mental illness; and that people suffering from severe mental illness may start using cannabis in order to alleviate psychotic, negative, affective, or anxious symptoms. This chapter will explore the scientific evidence regarding these hypotheses.

In addition, this chapter will examine consequences of cannabis use among people with mental illness. This will include a description of the self-reported reasons for cannabis use as well as a review of the scientific literature on cognitive function, therapy and medication compliance, symptom levels, utilization of mental health services, etc., among those dually diagnosed with cannabis abuse and mental illness.

Finally, a review of the existing treatment options for this type of comorbidity is explored. This will be based on a recent systematic review conducted by the chapter's author on people with schizophrenia spectrum disorders, but will be expanded to include other types of mental illness as well.

Chapter 2 - In recent years, cannabis potency and new methods for the drug's consumption have become heated issues. However, procedures for accurate measurement of cannabis consumption are still needed to assess the role of drug potency in rising rates of cannabis misuse disorders. This chapter presents a range of conceptual and methodological concerns related to accurately quantifying cannabis use. Analyses are based on a review of current literature on cannabis cultivation and markets and findings from a sample of 44 NYC-based consumers of cannabis. Subjects were interviewed about their drug use and, in some cases, observed consuming cannabis in natural settings. The findings indicate that using scales in the field to estimate cannabis consumption and attending to users' smoking methods, purchasing habits, and jargon for identifying different grades of cannabis are helpful tools for future research into the potential relationship between quantity, purity, and adverse mental and physical health consequences of cannabis consumption.

Chapter 3 - Cannabis remains an illegal substance according to the U.S. Federal Government despite some recent research suggesting that medical cannabis use is safe and has therapeutic potential for some vulnerable populations with chronic medical conditions. A public health perspective suggests that such legislation leads to increased health risks to vulnerable populations and potential reductions in quality of life. The APHA was one of the first American public health associations to formally recommend cannabis as an avenue for use in medical treatment and research. The following chapter discusses some of the main issues surrounding medical cannabis use among vulnerable populations from a public health perspective. A public health perspective suggests how such legislation may result to further increase disadvantage and health problems among vulnerable populations who are in need of alternative drug therapies. It is possible that legalizing medical cannabis has greater potential benefits than harms to vulnerable populations in the medical context who are not responding well to conventional treatment. However, realistic cautions should be taken to reduce cannabis dependence, potential respiratory problems, potential for accidents, or other undesired effects, and relatively safe means for cannabis intake should continued to be explored.

Chapter 4 - The goal of the present study was to explore the meanings of using drugs in adolescence and the relationship between these meanings and involvement in drugs. Participants were 208 adolescents (107 boys and 101 girls), aged 14-19 (mean age= 17.43, st.dev.= 1.55), attending two types of high school in Turin, Italy. Participants completed two questionnaires, one about involvement in drugs and other one about the reasons for having sex. Using confirmatory analyses, we found:

two dimensions of meanings for using drugs: Conformity and Self-affirmation, Coping; the Coping meaning was related to both higher involvement in drug use and habitual use of drugs;

The findings suggest some degree of similarity between meanings of using drugs and of heavy drinking. The findings also suggest that to reinforce the personal capabilities for facingstress and psychological discomfort might result in a more efficient strategy for preventing drug use with respect to other strategies; preventing substance use may also help for conforming to the behaviours of the other people and/or self-affirming one's own personality.

Chapter 5 - The consumption of Cannabis sativa held since 4000 BC being one of the first plants to be cultivated by man. Was recommend for prison-of-belly, malaria, rheumatism and also by adherents of some religions. Currently, marijuana is the most consumed illicit drug worldwide and the dependence is very common. In 2008, marijuana was used by 75.7 percent of current illicit drug users, in the USA. The effects and harm of marijuana use are well described and may involve physical effects such as tachycardia, dry mouth, dizziness, psychomotor retardation and psychological effects such as depersonalization, depression, anxiety, drowsiness and irritability. Chronic use complications can interfere with the operation of various systems such as pulmonary, reproductive and immune systems. The chronic user of marijuana may also submit amendments in relation to attention and the knee-jerk reactions. And these individuals may also report tolerance and withdrawal syndrome, as described in the literature. Marijuana is classified as a drug disturbing the central nervous system and its main psychoactive substance is the Δ-9-THC (tetrahydrocannabinol). After their consumption due to high lipid solubility, there is a change in the phospholipid membranes and the rapid action of THC on cannabinoid receptors. Few marijuana users seeking treatment for problem use of the substance and usually these individuals do not have the correct orientation of where to seek help. Pharmacological treatment for marijuana use and abstinence is not given and there are few studies on the subject. However it is known that psychosocial interventions are of great importance in the treatment to stop the use of marijuana.

Chapter 6 - In Italy the use of certain substances such as alcohol are encouraged and even guided by the family during adolescence, while others such as marijuana are strictly prohibited. Italian adolescents are among the highest in Europe for high-risk marijuana consumption. We investigated the one year longitudinal influence of our samples' personal (depression, stress, aggression, sensation seeking, and risk taking), family (strict family rule and parent approval of marijuana use), peer (peer approval of marijuana use and peer marijuana use) and school (academic marks) domains on three marijuana use indicators: lifetime use, past six month use frequency, and intoxication.

Research was conducted in the Italian province of Turin which is situated in Northern Italy. A sample of public high schools stratified by school type was invited to participate. The sample consisted of 324 youths (56% male) ranging in age from 15-20 (M = 17.29 yrs, SD = 1.61) living in northwest Italy and was reasonably balanced for gender (52% boys, 48% girls), and age (mean age = 17.4).

One year follow up analyses revealed that higher indications of depression at baseline were associated with lower indications of marijuana use at one year follow up ($\beta = -0.24$, $p = 0.03$), and with greater indications of marijuana use in the past six months ($\beta = 2.66$, $p = 0.004$). Similarly higher indications of sensation seeking at baseline were negatively associated with lifetime marijuana use at 1 year follow up ($\beta = -0.010$, $p = 0.008$). Higher indications of stress at baseline were associated with higher indications of lifetime marijuana use at follow up ($\beta = 0.14$, $p = 0.03$). Lastly, a greater perception of strict family rules at baseline was associated with lower indications of lifetime marijuana use ($\beta = -0.32$, $p = 0.005$) and with lower indications of past six month marijuana use frequency at 1 year follow up ($\beta = -1.54$, $p = 0.02$). Moderation analyses revealed a significant gender interaction between the association of sensation seeking and lifetime marijuana use ($\beta = 0.23$, $p = 0.004$).

This study represents a first attempt to uncover the marijuana use determinants of Italian adolescents. While not every important explaining factor has been studied here the authors have attempted to look at the effects of commonly studied adolescent marijuana use determinants in Italy. Continued efforts should be made to better explain both the risk and protective factors of marijuana use among Italian adolescents.

Chapter 7 - *Background*: Use of marijuana for both medicinal and recreational purposes has been linked to the stimulation of appetite and weight gain. Anecdotal observation of patients in a bariatric clinic indicated that this population engaged in marijuana use, despite their problems with weight management. The authors conducted a chart review to see elucidate the marijuana use patterns in a bariatric population.

Methods: A retrospective chart review was done on 20 patients. Marijuana use was identified, as well as the use of cigarettes, alcohol and other illegal drugs, as well as age of obesity onset.

Results: 25% of the patients used marijuana, which is higher that usage patterns for the general population (8.7%). Marijuana was not associated with use of other substances, or with age of onset of obesity.

Interpretation: The authors found a pattern of increased marijuana use in patients in a bariatric clinic. Further research is needed to better understand the nature of this finding and how it contributes to behavioral and pharmacological treatments of obesity.

In: Marijuana: Uses, Effects and the Law
Editor: Andrea S. Rojas
ISBN 978-1-61209-206-5

Chapter 1

MARIJUANA AND MENTAL HEALTH: ASSOCIATIONS, CONSEQUENCES, AND TREATMENT

Carsten Rygaard Hjorthøj
Psychiatric Center Copenhagen, Copenhagen, Denmark

ABSTRACT

Rates of cannabis use are consistently reported as much higher in psychiatric samples than in the general population, with some studies reporting abuse rates as high as 42 % among people with schizophrenia. This association has led to several hypotheses: That cannabis may be a causal agent in the development of schizophrenia; that cannabis may trigger schizophrenia in people who are vulnerable to the mental illness; and that people suffering from severe mental illness may start using cannabis in order to alleviate psychotic, negative, affective, or anxious symptoms. This chapter will explore the scientific evidence regarding these hypotheses.

In addition, this chapter will examine consequences of cannabis use among people with mental illness. This will include a description of the self-reported reasons for cannabis use as well as a review of the scientific literature on cognitive function, therapy and medication compliance, symptom levels, utilization of mental health services, etc., among those dually diagnosed with cannabis abuse and mental illness.

Finally, a review of the existing treatment options for this type of comorbidity is explored. This will be based on a recent systematic review conducted by the chapter's author on people with schizophrenia spectrum disorders, but will be expanded to include other types of mental illness as well.

The Marijuana – Mental Health Link

Rates of marijuana use have consistently been reported as higher among people with various psychiatric illnesses than in background populations. A systematic review of the existing literature on people with psychotic illnesses such as schizophrenia found that in this population, 23 % were current users, 29 % had used at some point during the last year, and 42 % had ever used cannabis. Prevalence rates for misuse were also high, with 11 % being current misusers, 19 % having misused cannabis within the preceding year, 22.5 % ever having misused [1]. A systematic review on patients with bipolar disorder found similarly high prevalence rates, with 22 % of the population being current abusers, and 36 % having a lifetime history of marijuana abuse [2]. Affective disorders such as major depression may also be associated with increased prevalence of cannabis use, however studies on the area have produced mixed results, as illustrated by a review from 2003 [3]. The review did show, however, a tendency to increased risk of depression among those who had used cannabis, though far from all the included studies showed this.

As detailed in chapter X of this book, these rates are somewhat higher than one would expect in the background population. The observation that cannabis use is more prevalent among people with psychiatric illness has given rise to a number of hypotheses that might explain this association:

1. Cannabis may be a causal agent in psychiatric illness
2. Cannabis may trigger psychiatric illness in those already disposed
3. Cannabis may be used by those suffering from psychiatric problems for purposes of self-medication

In the following, we will explore the scientific evidence regarding these hypotheses. In particular, we will emphasize on the link between cannabis and psychosis or schizophrenia, but will try to include other psychiatric illnesses as well.

Does Cannabis Cause Mental Illness?

The question whether cannabis causes mental illness is the classical question of causality. We know that there is an increased prevalence of cannabis use in people with a range of psychiatric illnesses. This does not necessarily mean, however, that cannabis has caused the mental illness in most or even just some of these people.

In a society where we would not have to worry about ethical issues, we could perform a randomized clinical trial (RCT) to establish whether such a causal link exists. This is used in many areas of biomedical research, and for good reason. The principle in an RCT is that you randomly assign people to one of two (or more) conditions, e.g. active treatment or placebo. When performed properly, this eliminates a number of problems that so-called observational studies suffer from. For instance, say we compare a group of people receiving one drug for cardiovascular disease with people receiving a different drug. We then observe a great difference in mortality between the two groups. The simple conclusion would be that one drug was much more effective than the other. If those receiving drug A had half the mortality of those receiving drug B, perhaps we should just give everybody drug A.

However, such inference could be wrong. For instance, it could very well be that drug B is given to a group of people that had no response to drug A, i.e. the most ill population. This is called confounding by indication. It could also be that drug A has more side effects that are not tolerated well in the elderly, so they instead get drug B. Elderly people are usually at a higher risk of dying than younger people, so perhaps the increased mortality in those receiving drug B was simply due to differences in age, not differences in treatment effect.

The above example is a good reason why we do RCTs. When it becomes completely random who gets which drug, then the only explanation you can find for differences in mortality would be differences in drug response. However, there are a great number of areas in which an RCT is not feasible, be it for ethical or practical reasons. For instance, it is often problematic to conduct RCTs in association studies. In the case of cannabis, it would probably be unethical to randomly assign people to, say, either use cannabis daily for ten years, or never use cannabis for ten years. It would also be impossible to control whether participants actually followed their assignment, without locking them up. So for areas such as exploring whether cannabis causes mental illness, other approaches than the RCT are required.

In 1965, the English epidemiologist Austin Bradford Hill proposed a set of criteria that could be used to judge whether an observed association would likely be of a causal nature or not. Most of them are not actual criteria, and not all of them need to be present before we consider some association to be causal, but they are a good guideline to go by.

1. Strength
2. Consistency
3. Specificity
4. Temporal relationship (Temporality)
5. Biological gradient (Dose-response relationship)
6. Plausibility (Biological plausibility)
7. Coherence
8. Experiment
9. Analogy (Consideration of alternate explanations)

At least one of the above is obvious, namely point 4 concerning temporality. The exposure must take place at an earlier time than the outcome. In our case, this means that cannabis cannot cause mental illness unless people smoked cannabis prior to the onset of the mental illness.

A number of studies have looked at the association between cannabis exposure and schizophrenia or psychosis while attempting to establish such a temporal relationship [4-8]. Some of these studies even attempted to control for psychosis-like symptoms in childhood. The reason for this was the idea that perhaps cannabis use could be caused by early, pre-clinical symptoms of mental illness. In general, these studies found an increased prevalence of psychosis or schizophrenia among those having used cannabis. A meta-analysis of the results indicated that the risk was increased by 40 percent among those who had ever used cannabis, and more than doubled in those who had used cannabis most frequently [9]. This does not mean that forty percent of cannabis users will develop a psychotic disorder such as schizophrenia. The forty percent increase is a relative risk, and is thus relative to the risk of developing such a disorder without using cannabis. The lifetime risk of schizophrenia in the background population is usually estimated at between 0.75 and 1 percent [10], meaning that heavy cannabis users might experience a lifetime risk of 1.5 to 2 percent – or higher, if they were subject to other known or suspected risk factors for schizophrenia. If this truly does constitute causality, it becomes possible to estimate the number of cases of schizophrenia that would be prevented if cannabis was no longer in use. For the United

Kingdom, with a population of about 15.5 million 15-34 year olds, around 800 annual cases might be prevented [11].

The meta-analysis mentioned above indicated the presence of a dose-response relationship between amount of cannabis consumed and risk of later development of psychosis. The findings of the included studies were consistent, thus fulfilling the third and fifth of Bradford Hill's criteria. It has also been suggested that criterion number six, that of biological plausibility, may be fulfilled, as the acute effects of cannabis in experimental settings are similar to those experienced during psychosis, e.g. paranoia, hallucinations and delusions [12]. Also, cannabis induced psychosis is a diagnosis available in the two major psychiatric classification schemes, namely the ICD and the DSM [13;14]. Whether the association is strong (criterion one) is debatable, and it would probably be both unethical and impractical to fulfill criterion eight and determine in an RCT if cannabis can cause psychosis. However, we are left with an impression that cannabis meets enough of the criteria for causality that we may consider it an indicator that a causal relationship could be inferred. We still need to consider alternative explanations, i.e. criterion nine. We will return to this a little later.

The meta-analysis by Moore et al. also reported on studies using affective disorders as an outcome. The overall result did show an increase in risk of such disorders (e.g. both unipolar and bipolar depression as well as suicidality); however, studies were more heterogeneous in their results and had fewer attempts at addressing non-causal explanations than was the case for psychosis. As such, the evidence for cannabis as a potentially causal agent in affective disorders is weaker than in psychotic disorders. Importantly, however, one should remember that *no evidence of causality* is not the same as *evidence of no causality*. In other words, the lack of an evidence base establishing proper temporal relationships in the association between cannabis use and affective disorders simply establishes that more and better studies should be conducted. By no means is there any indication that cannabis use *cannot* induce unipolar or bipolar depression.

The role of cannabis as a potential causative agent of other types of mental illness has not to this author's knowledge been examined. It does, however, seem unlikely that cannabis should be a direct cause of disorders such as PTSD, eating disorders, and personality disorders.

Does Mental Illness Induce Cannabis Use?

In the preceding section, we attempted to answer the question whether cannabis can cause mental illness, partially focusing on the temporal relationship of whether cannabis use came prior to the onset of mental illness. An alternative explanation for the association between cannabis use and mental health is the self-medication hypothesis. This hypothesis centers on the possibility that people experiencing symptoms of mental illness may use cannabis to alleviate these symptoms. Thus, the hypothesis is often referred to as a hypothesis of reverse causality. One indicator that this hypothesis may hold merit is that, when asked, people with psychosis often state that they use cannabis to alleviate symptoms, in particular negative symptoms (e.g. affective blunting, loss of interests or energy, etc.) [15].

One study has examined both possible timelines, i.e. cannabis use predating psychotic symptoms, and psychotic symptoms predating cannabis use [16]. The study found evidence for both relationships: Cannabis use, in individuals who did not have psychotic symptoms before they began using cannabis, predicted future psychotic symptoms; conversely, psychotic symptoms in those who had never used cannabis before the onset of psychotic symptoms also predicted future cannabis use. As such, without refuting what we found previously in this chapter, this study provided an interesting piece of information. Apparently, psychosis and cannabis use are so intertwined that introduction of one of these components increases the risk of the other being introduced at a later time. As we will see later in this chapter, consumption of cannabis may also lead to more pronounced psychotic symptoms. As such, it could be that the cannabis-psychosis duo functions as a sort of downwards spiral where it could even become futile asking whether the hen or the egg came first; regardless of what predates the other, the combination could spiral downwards to a set of undesirable consequences.

A review from 2003 also tested whether evidence supporting the reverse causality hypothesis existed concerning depression [3]. In other words, if depression could lead to cannabis use later on. The authors concluded that this appeared not to be the case.

Does Cannabis Trigger Psychiatric Illness in those already Disposed?

As we noted earlier in this chapter, the increased risk of psychosis resulting from cannabis use was only 40 % for ever users and 100 % for current misusers. As we also noted, this still meant that the vast majority of cannabis users would never develop psychosis. The fact that so many exposed persons do not develop mental illness has lead many observers to hypothesize that cannabis is more a trigger than a direct causal agent. Or, at least, that cannabis use is not *sufficient* for the development of mental illness. This leads to one final possible explanation for the cannabis-mental illness association; if a person is already disposed to developing a mental illness, the use of cannabis may be the triggering agent. This is akin to saying that exposure to cannabis interacts with something else, for instance genetics. This is often called a gene / environment (GXE) interaction.

The COMT gene has been hypothesized to have an influence on the association between cannabis use and psychotic symptoms. COMT is involved in metabolizing dopamine released into synapses. A mutation may generate a valine (val) to methionine (met) substitution at codon 158 of the gene. This means that three possible genotypes exist: val/val, val/met, or met/met. One study found that in people with the val/val genotype, adolescent cannabis users were 11 times more likely to develop a schizophreniform disorder than non-users; for the val/met genotype, the risk increased by a factor 2.5; and for the met/met genotype, no increased risk for schizophreniform disorder was observed among adolescent cannabis users [17]. Based on our earlier assumption that the lifetime prevalence of schizophrenia is about one percent, this means for people with the val/val genotype, upwards of 11 percent of those using cannabis during adolescence might develop schizophrenia. With approximately 25 percent of the population being homozygous val/val allele carriers, this constitutes a large subgroup of any population at significant risk of developing psychosis and schizophrenia if they use cannabis in adolescence.

In summary, it appears that cannabis may be implicated causally in the development of mental illness, in particular psychotic disorders such as schizophrenia, and possibly also affective disorders such as unipolar depression and bipolar disorder. Causality can sometimes also go the other way, as psychosis also increases the risk of commencing cannabis use. However, to this author's knowledge, little if any evidence exists that casts light on these relationships for other types of mental illness. In particular, it might be interesting to know what came first: increased prevalence of cannabis use on the one hand, and increased risk of PTSD, eating disorders, personality disorders etc. on the other.

Effect of Cannabis in Those Already Suffering from Mental Illness

As can be seen from the above, the exact nature of the relationship between cannabis and mental health can be difficult to disentangle. But one question is whether cannabis causes mental illness; another is whether cannabis can exacerbate an already existing mental illness. In trying to answer this question, we are faced with the problem of selection bias. For instance, if the literature suggests that among people with schizophrenia, those who use cannabis function better cognitively than those who do not, at least two explanations would be possible. One, that cannabis actually improves the cognitive capacities of people with schizophrenia, i.e. that had this group of comorbid cannabis users not used cannabis, their cognitive function would have been worse. Two, that schizophrenia causes such social and cognitive decline that only those with good cognitive skills are actually capable of having a misuse of cannabis. This is not merely a hypothetical situation as we are actually faced with this situation in a number of domains.

A number of domains have been studied, and here we will divide them into three groups: effects on cognition, effects on social skills, and effects on symptoms and healthcare utilization.

Cannabis Use in Mental Illness: Effects on Cognition

Several studies have shown inferior cognitive abilities associated with cannabis use in patients without psychiatric illness [18-20]. The effects are residual, i.e. not merely related to the acute intoxication. However, a recent meta-analysis on cognition in patients with schizophrenia and a history of cannabis use identified 10 studies and generally found the opposite tendency [21]. Cannabis appeared to be associated with improved cognitive abilities within a number of domains such as verbal fluency, executive functioning, verbal and visual memory, visuomotor speed, and face recognition [22-25]. Two of the included studies found no difference in cognitive abilities related to cannabis use [26;27], one found that cannabis use led to lower vocabulary scores [25], and one found that cannabis use led to worse performance in verbal memory and attention [28]. The latter article also investigated their own sample of first-episode patients and found that cannabis use was associated with improved visual memory, working memory, and executive functioning.

Generally, studies that looked at lifetime use of cannabis found improved cognitive abilities related to cannabis use, whereas studies looking at recent or current use found no such association. This may suggest a selection mechanism where a group of what the authors call “neurocognitively less impaired” patients only develop psychosis after a relatively early initiation into cannabis use. In particular, one study included in the meta-analysis found that earlier starting age of cannabis use was associated with better cognitive functioning [22]. Interestingly, another included study found a dose-response relationship where increased frequency of cannabis use was associated with better cognitive performance [25].

One study has looked at the acute effects of cannabis in schizophrenia. This randomized, double-blind study gave Delta-9-THC (the main psychoactive substance in cannabis) intravenously to 13 subjects with schizophrenia. Delta-9-THC was transiently associated with learning and recall deficits, as well as deteriorations on a number of non-cognitive domains such as psychotic symptomatology [29].

In view of the preceding findings, it seems unlikely that cannabis actually improves cognition in patients with schizophrenia in a causal manner. If it were so, the mechanism would be that acute intoxication of cannabis was bad for cognition, with this effect lasting until the category of “recent use”, where after a shift occurred and people having smoked cannabis were elevated to a higher level of cognitive ability than they started using cannabis. As such, the selection mechanism seems to be a more likely explanation.

The consequence of marijuana on cognition has not been well studied for most other mental illnesses. One French study on both psychotic and mood disorders also found improved cognitive abilities among those who abused cannabis [30]. This effect, however, disappeared when the authors adjusted for age, meaning that differences in age between abusers and non-abusers were the real reason for the observed difference in cognition. Using a slightly different approach, a recent study compared depressed cannabis dependents with non-depressed cannabis-dependents and found that those comorbid for depression scored better on some cognitive tests than did those with cannabis dependence alone [31]. A single study demonstrated improved cognitive performance in bipolar disorder among those with a history of cannabis use

[28]. Another study failed to find an effect of illicit substance use on cognition among patients with personality disorders [32]. A study in adolescents with ADHD found no difference in mean cognitive-perceptual score on the Schizotypal Personality Questionnaire between users and non-users of cannabis [33].

In summary, the effect of cannabis on cognition in patients with mental illness remains somewhat inexplicable. Taken at face value, cannabis seems to improve cognitive abilities within many types of mental illness. However, the mechanism is probably one of selection and confounding, with a group of "neurocognitively less impaired" patients only developing mental illness because they started using cannabis at a relatively early age.

Cannabis Use in Mental Illness: Effects on Psychosocial Measures

In non-psychiatric populations, cannabis use has been shown to be associated with poor psychosocial outcomes, such as poor economy, poor educational attainment, unemployment and other negative employment-related indicators, delinquency, and abortions [34-38]. It has also been pointed out that much of the effect disappears when controlling for competing, associated risk factors, leading to the possibility that the association may not be causal [39]. Contrary to what was expected, however one study found that among people with schizophrenia or bipolar disorder, both former and current substance abusers had a higher level of social functioning than did never users [40]. Quoting the authors, two domains of social role functioning were assessed: social and leisure functioning, reflecting the level of social activities and meaningfulness of interpersonal relationships; and instrumental role performance, reflecting the consistency and effectiveness of relevant role performance (e.g., worker, homemaker, student). The study did not, however, distinguish between alcohol, cannabis, and other illicit substances. A different study found that in treatment-resistant schizophrenia patients, those who abused drugs at baseline also had higher psychosocial functioning at baseline. [41] As both measurements were done at the same time (i.e. cross-sectionally), it is of course impossible to infer causality. Also, as is often the case, this study didn't distinguish between alcohol, cannabis, and other illicit substances.

One study compared psychosocial functioning between those comorbid for depression and cannabis dependence with cannabis-dependent patients without depression and found that comorbidity led to worse psychosocial functioning than did cannabis dependence alone [31]. This is a different approach than what has been looked at in the other studies mentioned, but does also provide at least some insight into the workings of comorbidity on psychosocial functioning.

In summary, little research has been performed on the psychosocial effects of cannabis use in people with mental illness. At least some of this research, however, indicates a protective effect of cannabis. As was the case for cognition, it cannot be ruled out that this indicates a selection or a confounding mechanism rather than a causal mechanism.

Cannabis Use in Mental Illness: Effects on Symptoms and Healthcare Utilization

Several studies have pointed out that in schizophrenia and psychoses in general, people who use cannabis (and other substances as well, for that matter) have reduced adherence to treatment, whether of psychosocial therapy nature or psychiatric medication [42-46]. To the extent that a treatment is beneficial to the patient, reduced adherence to the treatment regime must thus by inference lead to poorer treatment outcome and, probably, worse prognosis. One study found that reduced adherence to medication was prospectively associated with an increased risk of rehospitalizations, emergency room visits, homelessness, and symptom exacerbation [45]. Reduced adherence to treatment has also been shown to be associated with poorer quality of life, although the causality here can go both ways [42]. Cannabis-users may have reduced adherence to treatment for a number of reasons. As outlined previously in this chapter, acute intoxication and recent use of cannabis may lead to worse cognitive function, which could conceivably lead to reduced ability to follow the outlined treatment regime. Since cannabis use leads to more psychotic symptoms (see further along in this chapter), reduced adherence to treatment may also results from paranoid distrust of the psychiatrists, psychologists, etc. involved in treatment, and from reduced understanding of the fact that the patient actually has a mental illness. Additionally, it has also been suggested that cannabis may reduce the effect of antipsychotic medication, and vice versa.

Reasons for reduced compliance need not exclusively be a direct result of the effects of cannabis, however. The fault may also partially be found in the attitude of those who treat comorbid patients. One study has demonstrated that psychiatrists were significantly less likely to discuss the linkage between antipsychotic adherence and progress toward personal goals when facing a patient suffering from both schizophrenia and substance use disorder than when facing patients only suffering from schizophrenia. Conversely, psychiatrists were approximately two times more likely to add another antipsychotic for the group of comorbid patients [46].

General substance abuse [47] and abuse and dependence of cannabis in particular [48] have also been shown to increase risk of medication non-adherence in patients with bipolar disorder. Furthermore, it is known that poor adherence in this group of patients is related to lower remission rates [49] and less syndromal recovery [50]. Substance abuse is also shown to be associated with reduced compliance in unipolar depression [51-53], however to this author's knowledge, no studies have investigated whether the same tendency exists when looking solely at cannabis use disorders.

One study that made no distinction between type of psychiatric disorder found that of those with comorbid psychiatric and substance use disorder, 40.5 % were reported to have problems with treatment adherence [54]. The same study found that patients with adherence problems were significantly more likely to suffer from personality disorders than having other diagnoses. In contrast to this, one study indicated that among patients with eating disorders such as bulimia nervosa, the presence of substance use disorders does not predict treatment non-adherence [55]. A different study did find that abuse of psychoactive substances was associated with lack of adherence to cognitive behavior therapy, but conclusions can hardly be drawn from this study as it was based on merely six cases [56].

Whether related to adherence or not, patients with comorbid schizophrenia and cannabis use disorders are also at increased risk of rehospitalizations [57]. It has also been shown that a higher frequency of cannabis use predicted psychotic relapse in people with recent-onset psychosis [58;59], and this is apparently regardless of adherence to treatment and regardless of whether use of other illicit substances was present.

A follow-up study of people with recent-onset psychosis found a graded risk of positive psychotic symptoms at follow-up related to cannabis use. Compared with people who had not used cannabis at neither baseline nor at follow-up, those who had used cannabis at both time points had more than three times the risk of presenting positive psychotic symptoms at follow-up. For patients who had only used cannabis at one of the two time points, the increase in risk was smaller and not statistically significant from the null hypothesis of identical risk [60]. Another prospective study also found an approximately threefold increased risk of any level of psychotic symptoms in relation to baseline cannabis use [7]. The study also identified a more than twentyfold increase in risk of a severe level of psychotic symptoms, although the study was small enough that, due to statistical chance, the actual increase in risk could be anywhere from fivefold to more than hundredfold. Of further interest, negative symptoms of schizophrenia were not found to be related to cannabis use at baseline in the former study [60].

In summary, whereas the effects of cannabis on cognition and psychosocial measures in people with mental illness are debatable, there appears to be a strong effect on both adherence to treatment and illness-related measures in most types of mental illness. It is likely that for instance increased psychotic symptoms result both from the actual cannabis use and from the reduced adherence to treatment. Furthermore, while some psychotic symptoms are not always reducible through antipsychotic medication, their effects on anxiety and social functioning may be at least partially overcome through therapy, for instance cognitive behavior therapy. Since cannabis users also show reduced adherence to therapy, they may thus also experience more pronounced reactions to their psychotic symptoms.

Treating Cannabis Use Disorders in Mental Illness

As has been shown so far in this chapter, whether or not cannabis causes mental illness per se, there is good cause for treating cannabis use disorder in those already suffering from mental illness. The remainder of this chapter will focus on the evidence for different treatment strategies. At least two randomized clinical trials are still unpublished at the time of writing this chapter but will likely present results in the foreseeable future. The English MIDAS trial uses a psychosocial intervention combining motivational interviewing and cognitive behavior therapy for people with schizophrenia and any substance use [61;62], whereas the Danish CapOpus trial (which the author of this chapter is involved in) uses a similar treatment regime for comorbid schizophrenia spectrum disorder and cannabis use disorder (CUD) [63].

A Cochrane review of six trials [64-69] of psychotherapeutic interventions targeting CUD in people without comorbid psychiatric disorders pointed out that CUD is not easily treated [70]. A recent Cochrane review on psychosocial interventions for people with co-occurring severe mental illness and substance abuse disorder concluded that there was insufficient evidence to deem any one type of treatment better than others [71]. The latter review, however, did not focus on cannabis in particular. A systematic review published in 2009 and co-written by the author of this chapter attempted to focus on treating cannabis use disorders in people with schizophrenia spectrum disorders [72]. As such, it differed from the Cochrane review on several points, both by including only cannabis use and schizophrenia spectrum rather than the broader definitions of substance use and severe mental illness; and by focusing on any type of treatment and not just psychosocial interventions. Also, while the Cochrane review included only randomized trials, we included any type of study, though giving higher value to randomized trials of high quality.

We identified 11 articles treating cannabis as a separate outcome [73-83]. A further 30 articles were identified that explicitly included people with CUD, but where results were grouped together in a broader "substance use" category. Our findings were: contingency management (e.g. giving money to people for providing a urine sample without traces of cannabis) was effective, but the effect ended when the intervention stopped [81;82]. The two pharmacological trials treating cannabis as a separate outcome appeared effective, but neither was a randomized trial [79;83]. They both used antipsychotics (quetiapine and clozapine), and both drugs led to a reduction in cannabis use. However, since neither included a comparison treatment, it cannot be established whether the reductions were due to the medication or if they might have occurred regardless.

Psychosocial interventions were ineffective in most studies with cannabis as a separate outcome, including five randomized trials [73-78;80]. The trials compared different types of treatment. Two trials compared treatment as usual (TAU) with a combination of cognitive behavior therapy (CBT) and motivational interviewing (MI). Neither trial found one treatment to be better than the other [74;75], and one of them found no effect of either treatment [74]. A third trial found MI and psycho-education to be equally effective [76]. Surprisingly, one trial found TAU to be superior to MI [77]. However, the trial compared two sessions of MI with two sessions of TAU, and it may be argued that two sessions of MI are insufficient to be effective. The final trial compared to types of housing for comorbid homeless people, and a description of the contents of these types of housing is beyond the scope of this chapter.

In a secondary part of the review, we looked at the articles only reporting cannabis as a grouped outcome, i.e. with other substance and / or alcohol use disorders. Of note, psychosocial interventions, while ineffective in our primary review, were overall effective in this secondary review. In particular, both MI and CBT appeared to be effective in the secondary review [84-90]. The reasons for this are unclear, but one possibility is that interventions may have different effects on cannabis than on other substances.

The problem of grouped outcomes extends to other psychiatric diagnoses as well. A number of studies, e.g. many of those included in the aforementioned Cochrane review [71], simply look at a group of patients identified as having severe mental illness. They often also group cannabis together with other substances. Two studies conducted on patients with bipolar disorder failed to find an effect on illicit drug use, either overall or in comparison between the trial interventions [91;92]. However, though the articles provided separate data on cannabis at baseline, no such data or analyses were available for follow-up. To this author's knowledge, despite at least one study indicating substance being a poor predictor of treatment outcome for eating disorders [93], no trials have explicitly targeted the dual problem of eating disorders and cannabis use disorders. The same problem holds true for post-traumatic stress disorder (PTSD), with several studies only looking at substance use and not giving explicit data on cannabis. In general, these studies have found modest changes in substance use patterns over time, and generally without any one treatment proving more effective than any other [94]. One small trial investigating cognitive behavior therapy in adolescent girls with PTSD and substance use disorders did find better results on substance use outcomes in the therapy group compared with girls receiving treatment as usual [95]. While this trial also suffers from the issue of combining several substances into one, 78.8 percent of girls at baseline had a cannabis dependence diagnosis, and it can thus be expected that results will apply in particular to cannabis. The same intervention in a PTSD-substance use disorder population of incarcerated women did not, however, appear superior to treatment as usual, as both interventions caused the same improvement over time, again without separate figures for cannabis [96].

To summarize on the treatment of cannabis use disorders in mental illness, it must be concluded that as of yet, not enough empirical evidence to establish one any types of treatment as superior to others. Many trials include mixed types of substance abusers, without providing outcome figures for each type of substance separately. This may lead to the impression that one treatment is either effective or ineffective in general, but without providing information on the effect on cannabis abuse alone. Also, most studies have only looked at one type of intervention. To the knowledge of this author, no trials have looked at, for instance, combined psychosocial and pharmacological treatments of cannabis use disorders in schizophrenia. As such, we can finish this section off with a sentence so often used in systematic reviews and meta-analyses: *"More research is needed."*

Concluding Remarks

In this chapter, I have sought to outline the current state of knowledge on several areas related to the comorbidity of cannabis use disorders and other mental illnesses. The role of cannabis as a potential causative agent, perhaps as a trigger in those already vulnerable, has been established. It has also been established that cannabis use may result from psychosis, but not from depression. In addition, the effects of cannabis on cognition and on psychosocial functioning appear to be different in people with mental illness than in non-psychiatric populations. This is not likely due to a causally beneficial effect of cannabis, but rather a selection or confounding mechanism reflecting differences in mentally ill people with and without cannabis use disorders. We have seen that cannabis tends to exacerbate core symptoms of mental illness and to lead to reduced adherence to treatment. Finally, we have established that in general, we are currently unable to establish any one treatment for this sort of comorbidity as being superior to others.

There are certain aspects I have not looked into in this chapter. For instance, the fact that cannabis users often also use alcohol and / or other drugs is likely to influence some if not all of the associations outlined so far. People who use cannabis are generally also more likely to smoke tobacco. This leads to a number of possible interactions and confounding effects that may, if dealt with properly, alter some of what has been shown so far in this chapter. My reluctance to go into this area is in part based on the fact that relatively little existing empirical literature has dealt with it. However, studies that for instance exclude abusers of both alcohol and other illicit substances do generally come to the same conclusions as those who do not. As such, while going more into this might have further elucidated the subject matter, it may also have unnecessarily obscured many people's understanding thereof.

Another caveat to this chapter is that it has primarily focused on cannabis use in relation to psychotic disorders. This is not merely the fault of this author, however, as this simply illustrates the current state of knowledge on comorbidity research.

In order to give two final, concluding remarks, I would first like to echo the conclusion of the meta-analysis that looked at the potentially causal role of cannabis in psychosis: that while we may never have sufficient knowledge to *prove* that cannabis is harmful in relation to mental illness, we do currently have sufficient knowledge to *warn* that this is possibly the case; and secondly, that any researcher hoping to improve on the world's existing knowledge will find plenty of areas to improve upon in the subject field of comorbid cannabis use disorders and mental illness.

REFERENCES

[1] Green B, Young R, Kavanagh D. Cannabis use and misuse prevalence among people with psychosis. *Br J Psychiatry* 2005; 187(4):306-313.

[2] Cassidy F, Ahearn EP, Carroll BJ. Substance abuse in bipolar disorder. *Bipolar Disorders* 2001; 3(4):181-188.

[3] Degenhardt L, Hall W, Lynskey M. Exploring the association between cannabis use and depression. *Addiction* 2003; 98(11):1493-1504.

[4] Arseneault L, Cannon M, Poulton R, Murray R, Caspi A, Moffitt TE. Cannabis use in adolescence and risk for adult psychosis: longitudinal prospective study. *BMJ* 2002; 325(7374):1212-1213.

[5] Fergusson DM, Horwood LJ, Swain-Campbell NR. Cannabis dependence and psychotic symptoms in young people. *Psychol Med* 2003; 33(1):15-21.

[6] Henquet C, Krabbendam L, Spauwen J, Kaplan C, Lieb R, Wittchen HU et al. Prospective cohort study of cannabis use, predisposition for psychosis, and psychotic symptoms in young people. *BMJ* 2005; 330(7481):11.

[7] van Os J, Bak M, Hanssen M, Bijl RV, de Graaf R, Verdoux H. Cannabis use and psychosis: a longitudinal population-based study. *Am J Epidemiol* 2002; 156(4):319-327.

[8] Zammit S, Allebeck P, Andreasson S, Lundberg I, Lewis G. Self reported cannabis use as a risk factor for schizophrenia in Swedish conscripts of 1969: historical cohort study. *BMJ* 2002; 325(7374):1199.

[9] Moore TH, Zammit S, Lingford-Hughes A, Barnes TR, Jones PB, Burke M et al. Cannabis use and risk of psychotic or affective mental health outcomes: a systematic review. *The Lancet* 2007; 370(9584):319-328.

[10] McGrath J, Saha S, Chant D, Welham J. Schizophrenia: A Concise Overview of Incidence, Prevalence, and Mortality. *Epidemiol Rev* 2008; 30(1):67-76.

[11] Nordentoft M, Hjorthøj C. Cannabis use and risk of psychosis in later life. *Lancet* 2007; 370(9584):293-294.

[12] Murray RM, Morrison PD, Henquet C+, Di Forti M. Cannabis, the mind and society: the hash realities. *Nature Reviews Neuroscience 2007;* 8(11):885-895.

[13] WHO. International Classification of Diseases (ICD). http://www who int/classifications/icd/en/ [2008 Available from: URL:http://www. who.int/classifications/icd/en/

[14] Diagnostic and Statistical Manual of Mental Disorders DSM-IV-TR *Fourth Edition (Text Revision).* American Psychiatric Publishing, Inc.; 1994.

[15] Schofield D, Tennant C, Nash L, Degenhardt L, Cornish A, Hobbs C et al. Reasons for cannabis use in psychosis. *Australian and New Zealand Journal of Psychiatry* 2006; 40(6-7):570-574.

[16] Ferdinand RF, Sondeijker F, van der Ende J, Selten JP, Huizink A, Verhulst FC. Cannabis use predicts future psychotic symptoms, and vice versa. *Addiction* 2005; 100(5):612-618.

[17] Caspi A, Moffitt TE, Cannon M, McClay J, Murray R, Harrington H et al. Moderation of the effect of adolescent-onset cannabis use on adult psychosis by a functional polymorphism in the catechol-O-methyl-transferase gene: longitudinal evidence of a gene X environment interaction. *Biol Psychiatry* 2005; 57(10):1117-1127.

[18] Yücel M, Solowij N, Respondek C, Whittle S, Fornito A, Pantelis C et al. Regional brain abnormalities associated with long-term heavy cannabis use. *Arch Gen Psychiatry* 2008; 65(6):694-701.

[19] Solowij N, Stephens RS, Roffman RA, Babor T, Kadden R, Miller M et al. Cognitive functioning of long-term heavy cannabis users seeking treatment. *JAMA 2002;* 287(9):1123-1131.

[20] Grant I, Gonzalez R, Carey CL, Natarajan L, Wolfson T. Non-acute (residual) neurocognitive effects of cannabis use: a meta-analytic study. *J Int Neuropsychol Soc* 2003; 9(5):679-689.

[21] Yücel M, Bora E, Lubman DI, Solowij N, Brewer WJ, Cotton SM et al. The Impact of Cannabis Use on Cognitive Functioning in Patients With Schizophrenia: A Meta-analysis of Existing Findings and New Data in a First-Episode Sample. *Schizophr Bull* 2010;sbq079.

[22] Jockers-Scherübl MC, Wolf T, Radzei N, Schlattmann P, Rentzsch J, Gómez-Carrillo de CA et al. Cannabis induces different cognitive changes in schizophrenic patients and in healthy controls. *Prog Neuropsychopharmacol Biol Psychiatry* 2007; 31(5):1054-1063.

[23] Joyal CC, Hallθ P, Lapierre D, Hodgins S. Drug abuse and/or dependence and better neuropsychological performance in patients with schizophrenia. *Schizophrenia Research* 2003; 63(3):297-299.

[24] Stirling J, Lewis S, Hopkins R, White C. Cannabis use prior to first onset psychosis predicts spared neurocognition at 10-year follow-up. *Schizophrenia Research* 2005; 75(1):135-137.

[25] Schnell T, Koethe D, Daumann J, Gouzoulis-Mayfrank E. The role of cannabis in cognitive functioning of patients with schizophrenia. *Psychopharmacology (Berl)* 2009; 205(1):45-52.

[26] Sevy S, Burdick KE, Visweswaraiah H, Abdelmessih S, Lukin M, Yechiam E et al. Iowa gambling task in schizophrenia: a review and new data in patients with schizophrenia and co-occurring cannabis use disorders. *Schizophr Res* 2007; 92(1-3):74-84.

[27] Scholes KE, Martin-Iverson MT. Cannabis use and neuropsychological performance in healthy individuals and patients with schizophrenia. *Psychol Med* 2010; 40(10):1635-1646.

[28] Ringen PA, Vaskinn A, Sundet K, Engh JA, Jonsdottir H, Simonsen C et al. Opposite relationships between cannabis use and neurocognitive functioning in bipolar disorder and schizophrenia. *Psychol Med* 2010; 40(8):1337-1347.

[29] D'Souza DC, bi-Saab WM, Madonick S, Forselius-Bielen K, Doersch A, Braley G et al. Delta-9-tetrahydrocannabinol effects in schizophrenia: implications for cognition, psychosis, and addiction. *Biol Psychiatry* 2005; 57(6):594-608.

[30] Liraud F, Verdoux H. [Effect of comorbid substance use on neuropsychological performance in subjects with psychotic or mood disorders]. *Encephale* 2002; 28(2):160-168.

[31] Secora AM, Eddie D, Wyman BJ, Brooks DJ, Mariani JJ, Levin FR. A comparison of psychosocial and cognitive functioning between depressed and non-depressed patients with cannabis dependence. *J Addict Dis* 2010; 29(3):325-337.

[32] Taylor J. Substance use disorders and Cluster B personality disorders: physiological, cognitive, and environmental correlates in a college sample. *Am J Drug Alcohol Abuse* 2005; 31(3):515-535.

[33] Hollis C, Groom MJ, Das D, Calton T, Bates AT, Andrews HK et al. Different psychological effects of cannabis use in adolescents at genetic high risk for schizophrenia and with attention deficit/hyperactivity disorder (ADHD). *Schizophr Res* 2008; 105(1-3):216-223.

[34] Lynskey M, Hall W. The effects of adolescent cannabis use on educational attainment: a review. *Addiction* 2000; 95(11):1621-1630.

[35] Griffin BA, Ramchand R, Edelen MO, McCaffrey DF, Morral AR. *Associations between abstinence in adolescence and economic and educational outcomes seven years later among high-risk youth.* Drug Alcohol Depend 2010.

[36] Horwood LJ, Fergusson DM, Hayatbakhsh MR, Najman JM, Coffey C, Patton GC et al. Cannabis use and educational achievement: findings from three Australasian cohort studies. *Drug Alcohol Depend* 2010; 110(3):247-253.

[37] Schuster C, O'Malley PM, Bachman JG, Johnston LD, Schulenberg J. Adolescent marijuana use and adult occupational attainment: a longitudinal study from age 18 to 28. *Subst Use Misuse 2001;* 36(8):997-1014.

[38] Kandel DB, Davies M, Karus D, Yamaguchi K. The consequences in young adulthood of adolescent drug involvement. An overview. *Arch Gen Psychiatry* 1986; 43(8):746-754.

[39] Macleod J, Oakes R, Copello A, Crome I, Egger M, Hickman M et al. Psychological and social sequelae of cannabis and other illicit drug use by young people: a systematic review of longitudinal, general population studies. *The Lancet* 2004; 363(9421):1579-1588.

[40] Carey KB, Carey MP, Simons JS. Correlates of substance use disorder among psychiatric outpatients: focus on cognition, social role functioning, and psychiatric status. *J Nerv Ment Dis* 2003; 191(5):300-308.

[41] Buckley P, Thompson P, Way L, Meltzer HY. Substance abuse among patients with treatment-resistant schizophrenia: characteristics and implications for clozapine therapy. *Am J Psychiatry* 1994; 151(3):385-389.

[42] Coldham EL, Addington J, Addington D. Medication adherence of individuals with a first episode of psychosis. *Acta Psychiatrica Scandinavica* 2002; 106(4):286-290.

[43] Fenton WS, Blyler CR, Heinssen RK. Determinants of medication compliance in schizophrenia: empirical and clinical findings. *Schizophr Bull* 1997; 23(4):637-651.

[44] Kamali M, Kelly BD, Clarke M, Browne S, Gervin M, Kinsella A et al. A prospective evaluation of adherence to medication in first episode schizophrenia. *European Psychiatry* 2006; 21(1):29-33.

[45] Olfson M, Mechanic D, Hansell S, Boyer CA, Walkup J, Weiden PJ. Predicting Medication Noncompliance After Hospital Discharge Among Patients With Schizophrenia. *Psychiatr Serv* 2000; 51(2):216-222.

[46] Wilk J, Marcus SC, West J, Countis L, Hall R, Regier DA et al. Substance abuse and the management of medication nonadherence in schizophrenia. *J Nerv Ment Dis* 2006; 194(6):454-457.

[47] Gonzalez-Pinto A, Mosquera F, Alonso M, Lopez P, Ramirez F, Vieta E et al. Suicidal risk in bipolar I disorder patients and adherence to long-term lithium treatment. *Bipolar Disord* 2006; 8(5 Pt 2):618-624.

[48] Gonzalez-Pinto A, Reed C, Novick D, Bertsch J, Haro JM. Assessment of Medication Adherence in a Cohort of Patients with Bipolar Disorder. *Pharmacopsychiatry* 2010; epub ahead of print.

[49] Strakowski SM, Keck PE, Jr., McElroy SL, West SA, Sax KW, Hawkins JM et al. Twelve-month outcome after a first hospitalization for affective psychosis. *Arch Gen Psychiatry* 1998; 55(1):49-55.

[50] Keck PE, Jr., McElroy SL, Strakowski SM, West SA, Sax KW, Hawkins JM et al. 12-month outcome of patients with bipolar disorder following hospitalization for a manic or mixed episode. *Am J Psychiatry* 1998; 155(5):646-652.

[51] Zivin K, Ganoczy D, Pfeiffer P, Miller E, Valenstein M. Antidepressant Adherence After Psychiatric Hospitalization Among VA Patients with Depression. A*dministration and Policy in Mental Health and Mental Health Services Research* 2009; 36(6):406-415.

[52] Åkerblad AC, Bengtsson F, Holgersson M, von KL, Ekselius L. Identification of primary care patients at risk of nonadherence to antidepressant treatment. *Patient Prefer Adherence* 2008; 2:379-386.

[53] Akincigil A, Bowblis JR, Levin C, Walkup JT, Jan S, Crystal S. Adherence to antidepressant treatment among privately insured patients diagnosed with depression. *Med Care* 2007; 45(4):363-369.

[54] Herbeck DM, Fitek DJ, Svikis DS, Montoya ID, Marcus SC, West JC. Treatment compliance in patients with comorbid psychiatric and substance use disorders. *Am J Addict* 2005; 14(3):195-207.

[55] Agras WS, Crow SJ, Halmi KA, Mitchell JE, Wilson GT, Kraemer HC. Outcome Predictors for the Cognitive Behavior Treatment of Bulimia Nervosa: Data From a Multisite Study. *Am J Psychiatry* 2000; 157(8):1302-1308.

[56] Coker S, Vize C, Wade T, Cooper PJ. Patients with bulimia nervosa who fail to engage in cognitive behavior therapy. *Int J Eat Disord* 1993; 13(1):35-40.

[57] Caspari D. Cannabis and schizophrenia: results of a follow-up study. *Eur Arch Psychiatry Clin Neurosci* 1999; 249(1):45-49.

[58] Hides L, Dawe S, Kavanagh DJ, Young RM. Psychotic symptom and cannabis relapse in recent-onset psychosis. Prospective study. *Br J Psychiatry* 2006; 189:137-143.

[59] Linszen DH, Dingemans PM, Lenior ME. Cannabis abuse and the course of recent-onset schizophrenic disorders. *Arch Gen Psychiatry* 1994; 51(4):273-279.

[60] Grech A, van OJ, Jones PB, Lewis SW, Murray RM. Cannabis use and outcome of recent onset psychosis. *European Psychiatry* 2005; 20(4):349-353.

[61] Barrowclough C, Haddock G, Tarrier N, Lewis SW, Moring J, O'Brien R et al. Randomized controlled trial of motivational interviewing, cognitive behavior therapy, and family intervention for patients with comorbid schizophrenia and substance use disorders. *Am J Psychiatry* 2001; 158(10):1706-1713.

[62] Barrowclough C, Haddock G, Beardmore R, Conrod P, Craig T, Davies L et al. Evaluating integrated MI and CBT for people with psychosis and substance misuse: Recruitment, retention and sample characteristics of the MIDAS trial. *Addictive Behaviors* 2009; 34(10):859-866.

[63] Hjorthøj C, Fohlmann A, Larsen A-M, Madsen MT, Vesterager L, Gluud C et al. Design paper: The CapOpus trial: A randomized, parallel-group, observer-blinded clinical trial of specialized addiction treatment versus treatment as usual for young patients with cannabis abuse and psychosis. *Trials* 2008; 9:42.

[64] Brief treatments for cannabis dependence: findings from a randomized multisite trial. *J Consult Clin Psychol* 2004; 72(3):455-466.

[65] Sinha R, Easton C, Renee-Aubin L, Carroll KM. Engaging young probation-referred marijuana-abusing individuals in treatment: a pilot trial. *Am J Addict* 2003; 12(4):314-323.

[66] Copeland J, Swift W, Roffman R, Stephens R. A randomized controlled trial of brief cognitive-behavioral interventions for cannabis use disorder. *J Subst Abuse Treat* 2001; 21(2):55-64.

[67] Budney AJ, Higgins ST, Radonovich KJ, Novy PL. Adding voucher-based incentives to coping skills and motivational enhancement improves outcomes during treatment for marijuana dependence. *J Consult Clin Psychol* 2000; 68(6):1051-1061.

[68] Stephens RS, Roffman RA, Curtin L. Comparison of extended versus brief treatments for marijuana use. *J Consult Clin Psychol* 2000; 68(5):898-908.

[69] Stephens RS, Roffman RA, Simpson EE. Treating adult marijuana dependence: a test of the relapse prevention model. *J Consult Clin Psychol* 1994; 62(1):92-99.

[70] Denis C, Lavie E, Fatseas M, Auriacombe M. Psychotherapeutic interventions for cannabis abuse and/or dependence in outpatient settings. *Cochrane Database Syst Rev* 2006;(3):CD005336.

[71] Cleary M, Hunt G, Matheson S, Siegfried N, Walter G. Psychosocial interventions for people with both severe mental illness and substance misuse. *Cochrane Database Syst Rev* 2008;(1):CD001088.

[72] Hjorthøj C, Fohlmann A, Nordentoft M. Treatment of cannabis use disorders in people with schizophrenia spectrum disorders -- A systematic review. *Addictive Behaviors* 2009; 34(6-7):520-525.

[73] Addington J, Addington D. Impact of an early psychosis program on substance use. *Psychiatr Rehabil J* 2001; 25(1):60-67.

[74] Baker A, Bucci S, Lewin TJ, Kay-Lambkin F, Constable PM, Carr VJ. Cognitive-behavioural therapy for substance use disorders in people with psychotic disorders: Randomised controlled trial. *Br J Psychiatry* 2006; 188:439-448.

[75] Craig TK, Johnson S, McCrone P, Afuwape S, Hughes E, Gournay K et al. Integrated care for co-occurring disorders: psychiatric symptoms, social functioning, and service costs at 18 months. *Psychiatr Serv* 2008; 59(3):276-282.

[76] Edwards J, Elkins K, Hinton M, Harrigan SM, Donovan K, Athanasopoulos O et al. Randomized controlled trial of a cannabis-focused intervention for young people with first-episode psychosis. *Acta Psychiatr Scand* 2006; 114(2):109-117.

[77] Martino S, Carroll KM, Nich C, Rounsaville BJ. A randomized controlled pilot study of motivational interviewing for patients with psychotic and drug use disorders. *Addiction* 2006; 101(10):1479-1492.

[78] Nuttbrock LA, Rahav M, Rivera JJ, Ng-Mak DS, Link BG. Outcomes of Homeless Mentally Ill Chemical Abusers in Community Residences and a Therapeutic Community. *Psychiatr Serv* 1998; 49(1):68-76.

[79] Potvin S, Stip E, Lipp O, Elie R, Mancini-Marie A, Demers MF et al. Quetiapine in patients with comorbid schizophrenia-spectrum and substance use disorders: an open-label trial. *Curr Med Res Opin* 2006; 22(7):1277-1285.

[80] Shaner A, Eckman T, Roberts LJ, Fuller T. Feasibility of a skills training approach to reduce substance dependence among individuals with schizophrenia. *Psychiatr Serv* 2003; 54(9):1287-1289.

[81] Sigmon SC, Steingard S, Badger GJ, Anthony SL, Higgins ST. Contingent reinforcement of marijuana abstinence among individuals with serious mental illness: a feasibility study. *Exp Clin Psychopharmacol* 2000; 8(4):509-517.

[82] Sigmon SC, Higgins ST. Voucher-based contingent reinforcement of marijuana abstinence among individuals with serious mental illness. *J Subst Abuse Treat* 2006; 30(4):291-295.

[83] Zimmet SV, Strous RD, Burgess ES, Kohnstamm S, Green AI. Effects of clozapine on substance use in patients with schizophrenia and schizoaffective disorder: a retrospective survey. *J Clin Psychopharmacol 2000; 20(1):94-98.*

[84] Barrowclough C, Haddock G, Tarrier N, Lewis SW, Moring J, O'Brien R et al. Randomized controlled trial of motivational interviewing, cognitive behavior therapy, and family intervention for patients with comorbid schizophrenia and substance use disorders. *Am J Psychiatry* 2001; 158(10):1706-1713.

[85] Bellack AS, Bennett ME, Gearon JS, Brown CH, Yang Y. A randomized clinical trial of a new behavioral treatment for drug abuse in people with severe and persistent mental illness. *Arch Gen Psychiatry* 2006; 63(4):426-432.

[86] Haddock G, Barrowclough C, Tarrier N, Moring J, O'Brien R, Schofield N et al. Cognitive-behavioural therapy and motivational intervention for schizophrenia and substance misuse. 18-month outcomes of a randomised controlled trial. *Br J Psychiatry* 2003; 183:418-426.

[87] James W, Preston NJ, Koh G, Spencer C, Kisely SR, Castle DJ. A group intervention which assists patients with dual diagnosis reduce their drug use: a randomized controlled trial. *Psychol Med* 2004; 34(6):983-990.

[88] Kavanagh DJ, Young R, White A, Saunders JB, Wallis J, Shockley N et al. A brief motivational intervention for substance misuse in recent-onset psychosis. *Drug Alcohol Rev* 2004; 23(2):151-155.

[89] Kemp R, Harris A, Vurel E, Sitharthan T. Stop Using Stuff: trial of a drug and alcohol intervention for young people with comorbid mental illness and drug and alcohol problems. *Australas Psychiatry* 2007; 15(6):490-493.

[90] Martino S, Carroll KM, O'Malley SS, Rounsaville BJ. Motivational Interviewing with Psychiatrically Ill Substance Abusing Patients. *American Journal on Addictions* 2000; 9(1):88-91.

[91] Schmitz JM, Averill P, Sayre S, McCleary P, Moeller FG, Swann A. Cognitive-Behavioral Treatment of Bipolar Disorder and Substance Abuse: A Preliminary Randomized Study. *Addictive Disorders & Their Treatment* 2002; 1(1):17-24.

[92] Weiss RD, Griffin ML, Kolodziej ME, Greenfield SF, Najavits LM, Daley DC et al. A Randomized Trial of Integrated Group Therapy Versus Group Drug Counseling for Patients With Bipolar Disorder and Substance Dependence. *Am J Psychiatry* 2007; 164(1):100-107.

[93] Wilson GT, Loeb KL, Walsh BT, Labouvie E, Petkova E, Liu X et al. Psychological versus pharmacological treatments of bulimia nervosa: predictors and processes of change. *J Consult Clin Psychol* 1999; 67(4):451-459.

[94] Hien DA, Wells EA, Jiang H, Suarez-Morales L, Campbell AN, Cohen LR et al. Multisite randomized trial of behavioral interventions for women with co-occurring PTSD and substance use disorders. *J Consult Clin Psychol* 2009; 77(4):607-619.

[95] Najavits L, Gallop R, Weiss R. Seeking Safety Therapy for Adolescent Girls with PTSD and Substance Use Disorder: A Randomized Controlled Trial. *The Journal of Behavioral Health Services and Research* 2006; 33(4):453-463.

[96] Zlotnick C, Johnson J, Najavits LM. Randomized Controlled Pilot Study of Cognitive-Behavioral Therapy in a Sample of Incarcerated Women With Substance Use Disorder and PTSD. *Behavior Therapy* 2009; 40(4):325-336.

In: Marijuana: Uses, Effects and the Law ISBN 978-1-61209-206-5
Editor: Andrea S. Rojas

Chapter 2

WHAT'S IN A JOINT OR BLUNT?: METHODOLOGICAL CONCERNS IN THE MEASUREMENT OF CANNABIS CONSUMPTION

Luther Elliott*[*], *Andrew Golub and Eloise Dunlap
National Development and Research Institutes, Inc.
71 West 23rd Street, 8th Floor, New York, N.Y. 10010, USA

ABSTRACT

In recent years, cannabis potency and new methods for the drug's consumption have become heated issues. However, procedures for accurate measurement of cannabis consumption are still needed to assess the role of drug potency in rising rates of cannabis misuse disorders. This chapter presents a range of conceptual and methodological concerns related to accurately quantifying cannabis use. Analyses are based on a review of current literature on cannabis cultivation and markets and findings from a sample of 44 NYC-based consumers of cannabis. Subjects were interviewed about their drug use and, in some cases, observed consuming cannabis in natural settings. The findings indicate

---

[*] Corresponding Author. 564 46th St. Apt. 1, Brooklyn, NY 11220, Phone: 718-438-3970, Fax: 802-862-4685.

that using scales in the field to estimate cannabis consumption and attending to users' smoking methods, purchasing habits, and jargon for identifying different grades of cannabis are helpful tools for future research into the potential relationship between quantity, purity, and adverse mental and physical health consequences of cannabis consumption.

Keywords: Cannabis, Marijuana, joint, blunts, bongs, consumption intensity, field methods

INTRODUCTION

Between the 1990's and the early years of the new millennium, cannabis dependence rates rose sharply, particularly among young blacks and Latinos (Compton et al, 2004; NLAES, 2002; NESARC, 2006). Concerns over these trends have led to a number of speculative claims about the increased hazard of higher potency cannabis products and their potential role in problem cannabis use and related health consequences (McLaren et al, 2008). While chemical potency has long been considered an important variable in any study of substance use, this recent debate around cannabis potency and risk has highlighted the paucity of accurate data on cannabis consumption. Indeed, the National Research Council (2001, 75-123) has highlighted the need for systematic research on the topic of drug consumption.

> The absence of information on drug consumption leaves a major gap in the nation's ability to monitor the dimensions of drug problems. Data on drug consumption are essential to understanding the operation of drug markets; the dynamics of initiation, intensification, and desistance; the response of drug use to changes in prices; and the public health and economic consequences of drug use. *The committee recommends that work be started to develop methods for acquiring consumption data*. (NRC, 2001, *emphasis in original)*

Despite calls for data on drug purity and consumption there has been little information collected (see e.g., Johnson & Golub, 2007). Frequency of use remains an important indicator of the intensity of cannabis consumption in current research, but quantifying the amount of cannabis being consumed has been largely dismissed by researchers as unattainable (e.g. Budney et al, 1999). While acknowledging the difficulties inherent in accurate measurement of illicit substance use, this chapter presents methods for measuring key variables in cannabis use, including weight and potency.

MARKET DIVERSIFICATION AND NEW MARIJUANA

As some researchers began to observe around the turn of the new millennium, "new" marijuana markets have become increasingly diversified as designer or connoisseur-grade products have reached markets across the US (e.g. Schensul et al 2000). While there is no guarantee of higher potency therein, particularly as certain cannabis strains are highly desirable for their taste and smell, not their high potency (e.g., King 2006), local drug market trends toward higher average concentrations of cannabis' principal psychoactive cannabinoid, THC, are hard to dispute. John Walters, former director of the Office of National Drug Control Policy (ONDCP) argued in a number of major newspaper editorials that, "The potency of available marijuana has not merely 'doubled,' but increased as much as 30 times" (2002: D5). Although the potency of domestically produced and intensively cultivated cannabis has not been measured independently of lower-potency imported cannabis, a number of reports from the Netherlands, in particular, suggest that high-quality sensimilla distributed by cannabis cafes or medical cannabis boutiques is generally between 10 and 20% THC (EMCDDA, 2004; Ramaekers, 2006). This information is of central importance for cannabis researchers interested in the consumption or dosing practices of users. As a case point, two research participants each reporting use of a 500mg joint of cannabis could be in possession of as little as 25mg of THC in one instance and as much as 75mg in another. What goes unrecorded is the important fact that the first participant regularly consumes imported cannabis products grown in large fields and containing about 5% THC, while the second smokes an indoor-cultivated designer product with closer to 15% THC content.

Field researchers of cannabis consumption should, therefore, know how to ascertain cannabis quality by observation. Sifaneck *et al* (2007) have presented techniques for distinguishing designer versus commercial cannabis based on observable factors, such as density of glandular trichomes, color, and smell. Highly compressed plant material, for example, is a fairly reliable indicator of lesser quality bulk cannabis as is often imported from Central and South America. Other indicators of commercial cannabis include the presence of seeds and larger, "fan" leaves. Canadian export cannabis, largely from the province of British Columbia, has come to account for a larger market share in the US during recent years (Hurley et al 2010). It is generally considered to be of higher potency than imports from Mexico, Columbia, or Jamaica but not as desirable as designer domestic cannabis. Accordingly, Canadian export cannabis is generally much less expensive than domestic products that have not been packed for bulk shipment—a process that can result in a loss of fragrance and potency due to drying out and oxidation of THC-containing glands (e.g., Cervantes 2002). In one of the few studies to examine such differences, Sifaneck *et al* (2007) documented substantial differences in New York City street prices in 2005 ranging from around $8 per gram for lower-grade commercial to about $20 for high-grade designer cannabis. In other emerging research, analysis of stable isotopes in cannabis samples seized by police has been used to determine the characteristics of any particular sample of cannabis including whether it was grown indoors or outside and the country of origin (Hurley et al, 2009). This Marijuana Signature Project has effectively demonstrated the diversity of cannabis products available within any particular local market.

THC content appears to make a difference. Ramaekers et al (2006) have clearly demonstrated in the first clinical research to use medical-grade, intensively-cultivated cannabis, that executive and motor functioning are much more severely impacted by higher dosages of cannabis/THC. This said, it is clearly possible for consumers to control for this difference and modify their consumption behavior by titrating dosage. The data on this topic is limited to a few older studies with mixed findings. Perez-Reyes et al (1982) found that cannabis smokers do not alter their consumption when presented with stronger cannabis. On the other hand, Herning et al (1986) found they do. Both of these studies predate the widespread use of blunts, or inexpensive cigars in which the tobacco inside the wrapper or shell has been replaced with cannabis (Golub et al 2005). Further research on this topic is clearly needed given the importance of this topic and the broader changes in consumption practices in the last 25 years.

UNCERTAIN STANDARD UNITS

In addition to problems with measuring potency, the complex issue of quantity consumed also confronts research on cannabis consumption. First of all, cannabis products are generally sold to consumers in standard units of $5, $10, $20, and $50. However, the users often do not know how much cannabis, by weight, they receive when buying these “nickel,” “dime,” “dub,” or “cube” units, respectively (Sifaneck et al 2007; Harrison et al 2007). Harrison et al (2007) presented multi-site data from youthful drug markets using samples of 14-17 year old students, detained youth, and school dropouts in urban Philadelphia, Toronto, Montreal, and Amsterdam. Youth in the US and Canada mostly reported purchasing cannabis in nickel, dime or other small bags, which according to the authors varied substantially by weight. In Amsterdam, cannabis markets have greater standardization and purchasing experiences were very different. Dutch youth commonly reported quantities purchased in grams or joints (the units established in cannabis-selling coffee shops). The lack of standardization outside of Amsterdam, the authors conclude, "makes economic cost estimates suspect" in much extant research (ibid, S27).

The Impact of Interview Design

Adding to the uncertain relationship between frequency and quantity of use, survey methods themselves affect the ways users report quantity and frequency of cannabis use. There is extensive literature on survey design regarding measures of frequency and quantity in the field of alcohol research (e.g. Midanik and Hines, 1991; Midanik, 1994). These studies provide important lessons. Most centrally, the ways in which questions about substance use are posed tend to greatly affect the resulting responses. Blair et al (1977), for example, found that open-ended questions yielded nearly three times higher reports of past year alcohol use, compared with short or closed-ended questions (see also Bradburn et al, 2004). Others have argued that general questions about use in the past week, month or year produce less accurate results than questions that anchor use mnemonically to specific settings and contexts (e.g. Single & Wortly, 1994; Strunin, 2001).

Ascertaining Method of Administration

The staggering array of smoking methods available to the cannabis user today becomes immediately clear when visiting any head shop or tobacconist, either in person or online. From a perspective on cannabis consumption, the evident differences in smoking method are more than cosmetic. In a study of cannabinoid pharmacokinetics and pharmacodynamics, Grotenhermen reported that smoking a joint or blunt delivers 16-19% of the THC content of the cannabis to the mainstream smoke, with the rest lost to pyrolysis and sidestream smoke or left in the butt (Grotenhermen, 2003). The same study found that a pipe or bong (see figure 1.5) produces minimal sidestream smoke and yields up to 45% of the available THC to the smoker via the mainstream smoke. Vaporizing cannabis (rather than burning it) was assessed as delivering between 30 and 40% of the THC loaded into the device, just less than a pipe (Hazekamp et al 2006). To the best of our knowledge, however, no clinical work has examined in detail the pharmacokinetic implications of smoking pure cannabis (as is common in the US) versus smoking a blend of tobacco and cannabis or hashsish, as in the blunt or the European-style joint, cone, spliff, or blowtje (Sifaneck et al 2003). One study of New York City cannabis users found smoking blunts significantly increased the hazard of dependence (Ream et al 2008). Thus, for multiple reasons, the method of consumption serves as a variable as significant as potency in the study of cannabis related harms and is highly deserving of further research.

Social Contexts for Use

Perhaps the most grievous omission within current instruments used to assess cannabis consumption occurs when details about the social contexts for use fail to be elicited. Even where users are quite knowledgeable about quality and quantity dimensions of their use patterns, fundamental measurement problems can arise when cannabis is consumed in groups. Put simply, researchers and survey instruments that avoid investigation of the social contexts for use will tend to overestimate the intensity of when a participant reports consuming, for example, “four joints per day,” but is not asked to clarify whether those joints are shared or consumed alone. This issue is particularly salient in light of social conventions for smoking cannabis in groups (Dunlap et al 2005).

Aims of the Chapter

In light of these pressing concerns within scientific literatures and policy debates, this chapter presents findings from ethnographic research with 44 cannabis users in New York City in the interests of establishing preliminary strategies for collecting more accurate cannabis consumption data in survey and ethnographic field research. The scientific literature has not presented analyses of the range of consumption behaviors actually exhibited by cannabis users with respect to intensity of use. The preliminary findings presented serve to offer viable field methods where access to expensive techniques like gas chromatograph mass spectrometry (GCMS) and pharmacokinetic measurement devices are unavailable.

METHODS

Procedures

Participants for this project were recruited as part of a larger, longitudinal study of the contexts for use and abuse of cannabis, and particularly the cannabis blunt. Forty-four subjects participated in a follow-up interview in which they were asked detailed questions about their most recent episode of cannabis use. Ethnographers were trained to probe for information about the quality/type, quantity and dollar-value, and whether the cannabis in question had been shared among multiple parties. Rather than use the "joint" as a basic unit for measuring consumption rates as has been standard practice in national household surveys, ethnographers gained familiarity with a range of smoking methods and paraphernalia and urged participants to report on quantity, quality, and method of cannabis use in their own terms. Ethnographers also asked participants to describe the social, geographical, legal, and economic contexts for their use.

In addition to the survey data collected, two pilot investigations of smoking intensity and size of hits (or puffs) were conducted in natural settings expressly for preparation of this chapter. A long-time NY cannabis dealer and his female friend volunteered to carefully measure, prepare, and smoke a joint containing 300mg of high-quality cannabis. The researcher provided a scale that was accurate to .01 grams. The researcher instructed the subjects in a measurement protocol for weighing the joint after each turn. Each turn consisted of two hits in keeping with current conventions for social cannabis use often phrased as, "puff, puff, pass." After each turn, the joint was cleaned of any visible ash and quickly placed on the scale. The interviewer recorded the weight without touching the cannabis product. In this manner, the cannabis remained exclusively in the possession of the informant (see details of similar procedures in Sifaneck et al 2007). On another occasion, the experiment was repeated with the dealer and two other participants, this time smoking a blunt containing 700mg of another high-quality strain of cannabis. Blunts are typically much larger than joints.

Sample Characteristics

Potential subjects were recruited by participating in the life of various communities and by snowball sampling. The purposive sample included a diverse group of 44 participants, representing a broad spectrum of cannabis use profiles. Participants ranged from 15 to 62, with a mean age of 26. Fifteen were black/African-American, 4 Latino, 17 white, and 8 Asian-American. Subjects were primarily recruited from two very different locations. A sample of primarily university students and recent graduates was recruited downtown in Manhattan's East Village and Lower East Side. A sample of poor inner-city residents were recruited uptown, primarily in Harlem. Most of this latter group had not progressed beyond high school.

Participants were required to report having used cannabis in the past month. Frequency of use varied; 5 used less than once a week; 23 used multiple times per week; and 16 were daily users. There were definite racial differences in quality of cannabis used. Ten of the 15 white participants described consumption of higher quality cannabis compared to only 3 out of 19 for black or Latino participants. When asked about their familiarity with better quality cannabis, most Black and Latino subjects reported an awareness of designer strains, but indicated that they felt they were unable to afford them. Door, a 37-year-old Black woman, offered a typical response when asked about popular designer strains:

> *Q:* So you don't know about types like chronic and...purple haze and hydro and all that?
>
> *Door:* I know about them but um, that's a little out of my budget.

As with Door, all of the study participants quoted below are referred to by the pseudonyms (but not real street names) they created for themselves for exclusive use by this project.

RESULTS

Marketplace Diversity and Homogeneity

Even without the benefit of first-hand observations of the cannabis being used by study participants, researchers can use market information to elicit an estimate of the quality of cannabis consumed. When asked to describe, in their own terms, the quality of cannabis that they smoke, our participants alternated between market labels and more informal quality descriptors. Price data, when available, provides another indicator. This information usually can distinguish whether participants are using a commercial or designer product.

Those in our sample accustomed to smoking less-expensive, imported cannabis often referred to the quality of the cannabis they smoked as regular, mediocre, decent, or plain weed. Imported cannabis that proved unsatisfactory to the consumer was referred to as dirt weed, garbage, or crap. Complicating matters somewhat at the low end of the quality spectrum, a number of participants referred to the relatively inexpensive cannabis they smoke using market labels such as Arizona and Chocolate (Johnson et al 2005). While the branding of cannabis as such might suggest a higher quality domestic product, the samples designated as such in Sifaneck et al (2007) clustered around the lower end of the price spectrum and were hypothesized to originate from Mexico and Jamaica, respectively. Several of our ethnographic participants reporting use of either Chocolate or Arizona made the same point, as in the following from 26-year-old black American female, Taylor:

> I think they make those names up just to make it sound good sometimes. I'm serious...All that Chocolate, because it's brown...I have no idea how to tell one from another.

While no study participants referred explicitly to Canadian cannabis in their accounts, a number described what was likely Canadian "mids," a term used for mid-grade cannabis by users, dealers, and consumer-driven market indices such as *High Times*' Trans High Market Quotes (http://hightimes.com/tags/thmq). Seventeen-year-old high school student, Snake, describes cannabis somewhere in the middle of the quality/potency spectrum:

> Um, it was like Hydro. It was like no seeds or anything. It was like-it wasn't too great. But it wasn't bad.

Using the term, "skunk," another catch-all for designer cannabis potentially derived from one of the early high-potency cannabis hybrids that bore a strong skunk-like odor, a 20-year-old black college student, Triple A, describes the cannabis he consumed:

> It wasn't like Blueberry or anything but it was effective... . It was Skunk but it didn't have like a lot of crystals or anything on it.

For experienced cannabis users with whom we spoke, the density of the trichome "crystals" evident on cannabis flowers (or "buds") and leaflets served as one of the most reliable indicators of cannabis potency available to the consumer. Cannabis growers and connoisseurs have reported using microscopes to examine in forensic detail the maturity and density of glandular trichomes. The electronics chain retailer, Radio Shack, offers a popular hand-held microscope for $10.99. Of the 43 reviews posted on Radio Shack's website as of July 1, 2010 (www.radioshack.com/sm-see-all-needs-and-wants--pi-2179604.html), 16 make explicit reference to trichomes or trichs for short. Although use of microscopes in the field will never provide accurate measures of THC content in a cannabis sample, the tool may nonetheless prove valuable to researchers wanting to strengthen their ability to use plant anatomy as an indicator of the grades and potencies of cannabis being consumed by study participants. Particularly where cannabis has been centrifuged (see: www.pollinator.nl) or treated roughly during drying and packaging for export, capitate-stalked trichomes, as pictured in Figure 1.1, will often appear matted, or as straight stalks lacking in the large bulbous glands depicted below.

Users of designer cannabis were far more likely to use brand-names as a means of describing their recent purchases and consumption. Ideally, the marketing labels given to cannabis would follow directly from the breeders and can be referenced via such recent photographic compendia as *The Big Book of Buds* (Rosenthal & Newhart 2001; 2004) or seed clearinghouses like www.seedbay.com. As many of our participants indicated, however, the brand names actually circulating are often coined by middlemen and dealers themselves, in the interests of up-marketing lower-quality cannabis (Johnson et al 2005).

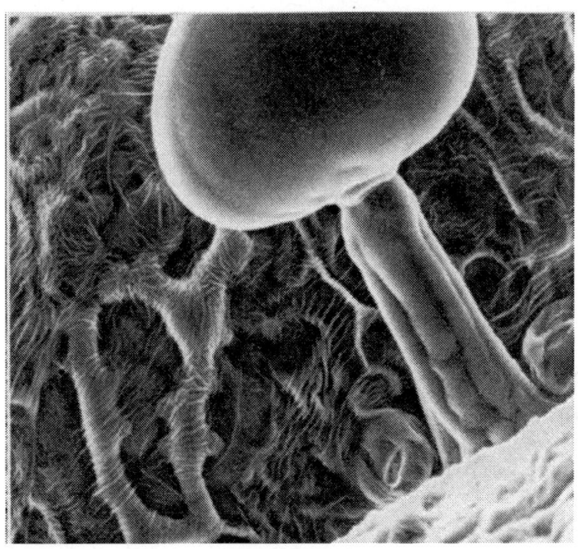

Figure 1.1. Cannabis glandular trichome (400X), reprinted from Dayanandan & Kaufman (1976).

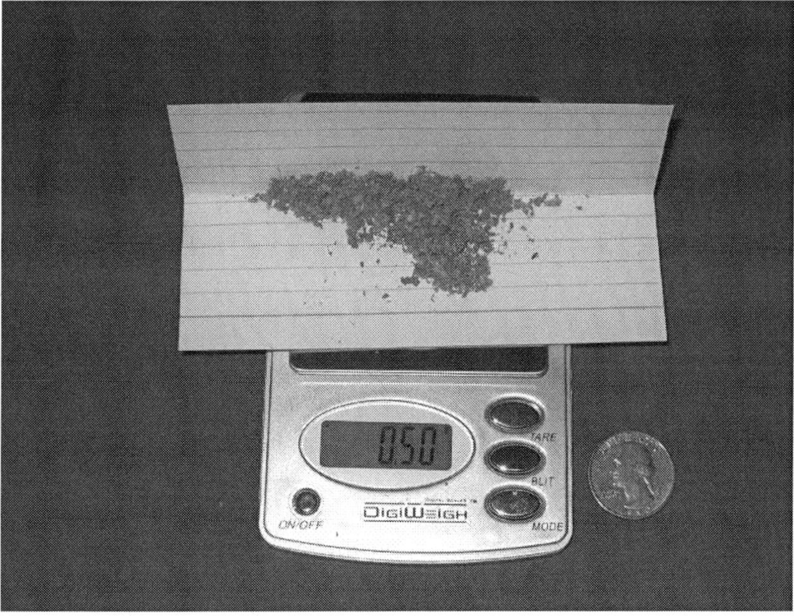

Figure 1.2. The contents of a "standard" joint: .5g of designer marijuana cut for rolling. Photo by lead author.

With the number of marketable strains available to the contemporary grower increasing every year, and the potential for creative renaming of products at every step along the supply chain, it is clearly impossible for the cannabis researcher to become an expert in identifying or verifying the exact pedigree of any given cannabis sample. On the other hand, any such efforts could well pay off in most research contexts. Even within a metropolis as large as NYC, a small number of recognizable strains appeared to dominate the high-end market during the timeframe for this research (Sifaneck et al, 2005). For that subset of cannabis users reporting recent use of high-quality cannabis in this study, the most commonly used designer variety was "haze," a label which has been in existence since the 1970's when the hybrid was allegedly developed in California (e.g., King 2006). Known to be a predominantly *cannabis sativa* hybrid with extremely long flowering times and large plant size, haze is generally referred to as an outdoor strain largely unsuited to today's greenhouse and grow-room environments (ibid). In keeping with this botanical profile, project ethnographers heard several stories circulating in NYC about a large outdoor cannabis operation in Florida swamps producing the bulk of the haze commercially available through youthful Dominican commercial networks during recent years.

Standard Consumption Units—Joints

Although illicit drug research has always lacked the equivalent of alcohol research's standard unit, the joint has long served as the means of estimating quantity of use for those studies that even attempt it. While the joint remains an almost universally recognized unit of cannabis consumption, several problems with the joint as a benchmark unit of analysis in drug abuse research have been raised during the course of this study and likely relate to changing trends in use of designer cannabis and/or distinct regional differences in the preparation of cannabis for consumption.

First, interviewees using the cannabis joint as their favored delivery mechanism presented varying quantities when asked how much cannabis they commonly use in rolling a joint. All of our regular joint smokers indicated use of less than half a gram per joint, the current norm on survey instruments (see fig. 1.2). Indeed, regular purchasers described making two to three joints from each "nickel [bag]" ($5) purchase of cannabis. Sifaneck *et al* (2007) found that the average weight of cannabis sold in $5 units in NYC during the period of research was 0.75g. Thus, the modal joint in this study weighed less than 0.35

grams, and probably even less given that larger stems and any seeds would have been removed, further reducing the quantity of consumable cannabis in any commercial-grade purchase. One experienced, 43-year-old cannabis smoker in our work referred to the actual weight of a joint, independent of any retail unit, when asked how much cannabis he used in a recent use episode:

> *Jerry:* Maybe point three [.3 grams]. That's what is considered to be in a joint.
> *Q:* Was it a skinny joint, a fat joint, or what?
> *Jerry:* Just a regular joint.

For other users, joints are simply not an appropriate frame of reference for their typical smoking patterns, because they do not typically smoke joints. Some referred to joints as "old school" and as the method preferred by "old-timers." Many stated clear preferences for smoking blunts.

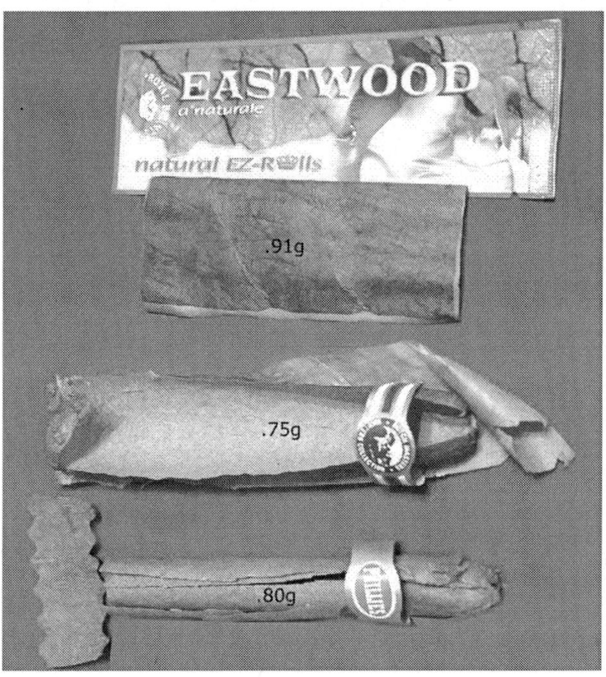

Figure 1.3. Control Weights for Blunt "Wraps" and Cigars prepared for Blunt manufacture. From top to bottom: Eastwood natural flavored blunt 'wrap,' Dutch Masters cigar shell and binder, Philles Blunt cigar shell and binder with "cancer piece" removed (left). Photo by lead author.

Standard Consumption Units—Blunts

In recent years, the blunt has become a popular alternative to pipes and joints, especially among black youths (e.g. Golub et al 2005; Sifaneck et al 2005). Even more than the joint, the quantity of cannabis in a blunt appears to be determined by the amount contained in standard retail purchases of $5 and $10 of cannabis. Seventeen of 44 participants reported smoking cannabis blunts as their preferred method for smoking cannabis. All but two of the 17 reported using one nickel bag of cannabis in the construction of a standard blunt. Both of the accounts of using larger quantities involved $10 quantities of cannabis. For one user, a blunt (with $10 of "regular" cannabis) was intended for sharing among a larger group. For the other, $10 of designer cannabis (about a half gram) constituted a standard preparation for unshared personal consumption.

RIZLA+
.05g
ZIG-
ZAG 1¼
.06g
Bambu
.08g
Smoking
.08g
e-z wider
Double
Wide
.11g

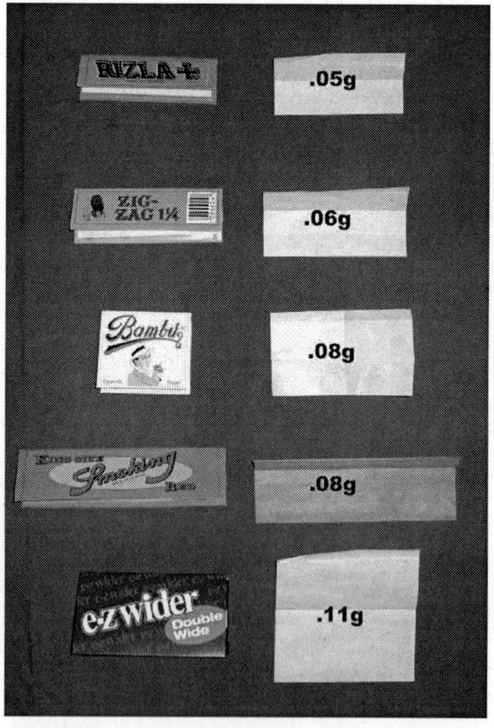

Figure 1.4. Control Weights for Popular Cigarette Papers. From Top to Bottom: Rizla, Zig-Zag (1 ¼), Bambu, King Size Smoking, E-Z Wider (Double Wide). Photo by lead author.

Standard Consumption Units—Bowls and Bongs

Use of cannabis pipes in the US has changed considerably since the late-1960s. Judging from our informants' accounts corn cob and clay pipes and inexpensive "bowls" made of copper and aluminum plumbing apparatus have largely given way to blown glass paraphernalia. Water pipes, or "bongs," as well have seen considerable technological developments. Although inexpensive vinyl versions with aluminum metal "slide" pieces are still widely available, the current trend is again toward glass and, in particular, heavy laboratory-grade Pyrex™. A 36-year-old male cannabis dealer in the study, DJ Charisma, volunteered to bring a range of paraphernalia to an interview session, including the glass bong depicted in figure 1.5. Though the "tube" itself is simple and cost only $140, he explained, he purchased the "ash catcher" attachment and colorful hand-blown bowl separately which brought the total to $250. Top brands like Roor, Amsterdam Design Studios, Jerome Baker Design, and Illadelph can easily command prices between $250 and $500 without any add-ons, making the glass bong one of the most high-status cannabis consumption mechanisms (see, e.g., www.roor.de).

While the bong is often spoken of as a filtration device, providing cooler and less tar-rich smoke, its reputation among our informants was complicated by its apparent associations both with affluent whites and extreme cannabis intoxication. Discussing their preferences for joints or blunts, a number of interviewees speak of the bong as an expensive and inflexible apparatus with no utility beyond the home. Twenty-five-year-old female secretary M. Norwood states her preference for less obtrusive smoking methods, and suggests that public displays of a bong are inconceivable, "unless you're like a dorky college student or something. You want to play hacky-sack outside and smoke your bong [laughs]." For one of the daily blunt users in the study, the bong is described as simply "too much." Asked to clarify, the 20-year-old African-American grocery store worker, Packer, explains: "Like when you smoke out of a bong…you put more in your lungs than what comes out."

Due to the contradictory reports of the bong's specific benefits and utility, the bong can present considerable difficulties for research into the probable dosage of cannabis smoke being consumed. Perhaps the most important distinction to be made is whether users are smoking the entire quantity of cannabis loaded into the "slide" or bowl piece in one large draw or "hit," or whether the bong is shared or smoked over several episodes. Like the pipe (or "bowl") depicted in figure 1.6, standard bong "slides" typically hold between 150 and 300mg of cannabis. Unlike pipes, bongs present the possibility of smoking very rapidly and inhaling very deeply, leading to high levels of intoxication and higher absorption of THC and tar, as Packer alludes to above.

This research has identified strong conventions governing the number of hits to be taken from joints and blunts before passing to another consumer. "Puff, puff, pass" is the popular colloquial phrasing of the two-hit rule for social smoking. The social etiquette and standard conventions for bong use are far less studied. One qualitative investigation of smoking methods in France found that bong users "described specific physical risks such as respiratory problems and fainting" and that the bong's "sudden and violent effects put cannabis in league with hard drugs" (Chabrol et al, 2004). Clearly this conception of the bong might serve to draw different social boundaries around bong users. Research of this nature has not been conducted in the US, however, where smoking a bong would appear far more likely to involve pure cannabis, rather than a mixture of cannabis and tobacco.

Quantifying the "Hit"

For users to report accurately on the amount of cannabis smoked during an episode, it is frequently necessary to subdivide standard consumption units to account for shared use or for the conservation of some portion of the cannabis contained in a joint, bowl, bong, or blunt. Since many participants referred to smoking "clips" or "roaches" (i.e. the extinguished remains of a joint or blunt), the number of "puffs" or "hits" taken during an episode is often the most reliable indicator of quantity that informants can provide. Particularly when participants are infrequent users or are otherwise unaware of the amount of cannabis prepared by a peer for a joint, blunt, or pipe, the number of hits the participant recalls taking him/herself can be a valuable measure for researchers.

Two pilot investigations provide working guidelines for estimating the amount of cannabis consumed in a hit. In experiment 1, two participants, a 35 year-old male and a 29 year-old female, carefully prepared a joint containing 300mg of high-quality cannabis. The cannabis was reported to be Strawberry Cough, a popular strain bred in the Netherlands by Dutch Passion (see: http://www.dutch-passion.nl) and being sold by the male participant, a longstanding cannabis dealer, for $450/oz. The results of the consumption episode are presented in Table 1. It was estimated that a hit involved about 10 milligrams of cannabis, after accounting for paper weight and the discarded roach. One preliminary finding is that a more precise scale could be used for measuring the size of a hit. The .01 gram accuracy was barely sufficient for our calculations.

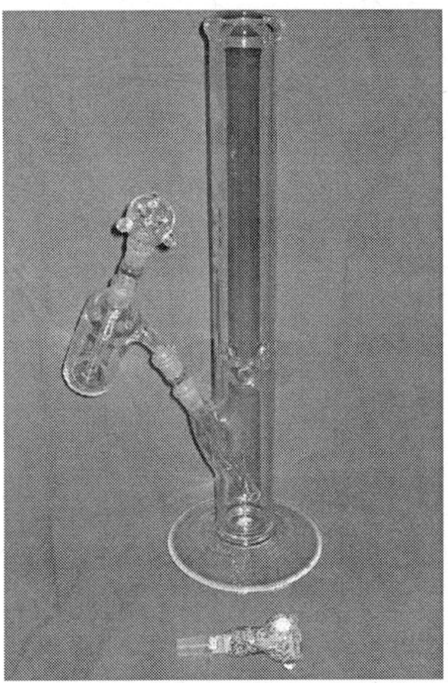

Figure 1.5. High-status smoking: A glass "bong" with "ash-catcher" and extra "slide." Photo by lead author.

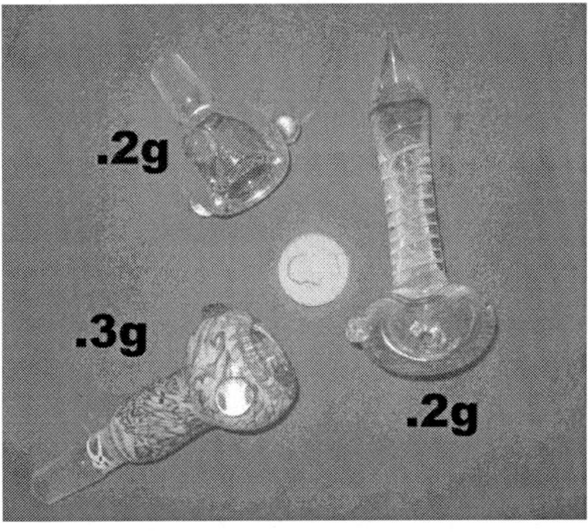

Figure 1.6. Bong "slide" (left) and glass "bowl" capacities. Photo by lead author.

Table 1. Quantity (gm) of cannabis per hit from one high-potency joint

Turn #[a]	Weight of joint after turn	Change in weight	Size of hit[b]
0[c]	0.36		
1 (♂)	0.32	0.04	0.016
2 (♀)	0.29	0.03	0.012
3 (♂)	0.27	0.02	0.008
4 (♀)	0.24	0.03	0.012
5 (♂)	0.22	0.02	0.008
6 (♀)	0.20	0.02	0.008
7 (♂)	0.17	0.03	0.012
8 (♀)	0.14	0.03	0.012
9 (♂)	0.12	0.02	0.008
10 (♀)	0.10	0.02	0.008
11 (♂)	0.08	0.02	0.008
12 (♀)	0.06	0.02	0.008

[a] Participants took the standard two hits per turn.
[b] This includes a correction of .79 for the paper and .50 for taking two hits per turn.
[c] Prior to being lit.

In the blunt smoking episode, the male dealer prepared a blunt with his preferred cigar, the Dutch Masters Corona (see fig 1.3). This time the cannabis used was White Widow, another Dutch Passion strain, listed on the company's website as having a potency estimate of 18.9% THC; this product appeared to have more intact glandular trichomes than the Strawberry Cough sample used in the joint measurement. At $475/oz, the 700mg quantity of cannabis used to make a blunt representative (in quantity and size) of the modal blunt for the ethnographic sample would cost the user roughly $13, including the $1.25 cigar. Purchased in smaller quantities, the same cannabis might cost considerably more and push the cost of a single designer blunt up to $20.

Controlling for the weight of the cigar binder and wrapper used in the blunt required several additional corrections, compared with the standard joint. Although the initial weight of the Dutch Masters Corona emptied of its filler was measured at 850mg (see figure 1.3), a number of modifications were made to the binder and wrapper in the process of rolling the blunt. After moistening the tapered mouth end of the cigar and carefully unrolling the leaf wrapper, the male dealer proceeded to split the underlying binder along its gummed seam with his thumbnail. Carefully folding back this ½" margin where the binder overlaps, he then tore it off, explaining that the gummed strip provides an undesirable and unhealthy "heaviness" to the smoke as well as a cumbersome amount of width on the binder, which he and others in our research have referred to as the "cancer paper." In the final step before rolling, the scalloped paper layer lying between the wrapper and the binder at the mouth end of the cigar, or "cancer piece" (see Schensul et al 2000) was also removed. Once rolled, the blunt often undergoes even further adjustments, as the cannabis at both ends of the refashioned cigar is often less densely packed than in the middle and needs to be tamped, in this case with the cap of a ball-point pen. This technique allows one or both ends of the blunt to then be trimmed or burnt off and, in this instance, produced a completed blunt weighing 1.10 grams. As no cannabis was lost in the preparation of the blunt, the total weight of cigar product in the final product was 0.4g, giving a cannabis to cigar ratio of 7:4 (i.e. ~64% cannabis; ~36% cigar product). The results of this blunt sharing episode are presented in Table 2.

Table 2. Quantity (gm) of cannabis consumed per hit from one high-potency blunt

Turn #[a]	Weight of joint after turn	Change in weight	Size of hit[b]
0[c]	1.10		
1 (♂$_1$)	1.04	0.06	0.019
2 (♀)	0.94	0.10	0.032
3 (♂$_2$)	0.87	0.07	0.022
4 (♂$_1$)	0.78	0.09	0.029
5 (♀)	0.71	0.06	0.019
6 (♂$_2$)	0.66	0.05	0.016
7 (♂$_1$)	0.58	0.08	0.026
8 (♀)	0.53	0.05	0.016
9 (♂$_2$)	0.46	0.07	0.022
10 (♂$_1$)	0.41	0.05	0.016
11 (♀)	0.37	0.04	0.013
12 (♂$_2$)	0.32	0.05	0.016
13 (♂$_1$)	0.27	0.05	0.016

[a] Participants took the standard two hits per turn.

[b] This includes a correction of .64 for the cigar wrapper and .50 for taking two hits per turn.

[c] Prior to being lit.

Results from the blunt smoking experiment indicate a considerably larger average hit than with the joint. After controlling for the cigar shell, the mean hit was just above 20mg, or roughly double the mean hit size from a joint made with 300mg of cannabis. Thus, while weighing roughly 700mg more than the joint used in the earlier experiment, the blunt provided only 2 more hits (26 vs 24) than the joint. The largest 2-hit turn in the experiment was taken by the female participant, who then had an intense coughing episode and acknowledged her preference for joints. During her next 3 turns (numbers 5, 8, and 11 on Table 2), however, she corrected her technique to avoid further coughing and took considerably smaller draws. After all 3 participants agreed that they were sufficiently high, the remaining "clip" was extinguished, left in the ash tray, and designated as a "pick-me-up" for later use.

Calculating THC Consumed

The information presented in this paper provides enough information for a rough estimate of the amount of cannabis consumed in the two episodes described above using the following formula:

$$\begin{bmatrix} THC \\ Consumed \end{bmatrix} = \begin{bmatrix} Weight \\ of\ Cannabis \end{bmatrix} \times \begin{bmatrix} Potency \\ \end{bmatrix} \times \begin{bmatrix} \%\ available\ by \\ Smoking\ method \end{bmatrix}$$

In the joint smoking session, both the male and female participant consumed approximately 0.12g of Strawberry Cough cannabis. Based on quality indicators discussed above, such as strain name, appearance, and price paid (per gram), a reasonable estimate of cannabis potency would be about 15% THC for the carefully cultivated, designer sensimilla consumed (see also Gieringer 1999). Grotenhermen's figures indicate that smoking in a rolled product transfers a maximum of about 19% of the THC available. Putting it all together yields an estimated dose of 3.4mg (0.12g × 0.15 × 0.19) of THC consumed by each of the participants.

In the blunt smoking episode, the first male participant consumed roughly 0.21g of White Widow, while the female and second male participants consumed about 0.15g each. Again, this is a high quality cannabis product and the expected available THC from smoking would be about 19%. The formula yields estimates of 7.5mg for the first participant and 5.4mg for the others.

Discussion

Accurately quantifying drug consumption rates for an illegal, unregulated, and highly variable plant substance can involve expensive and awkward equipment.. The most precise setup would involve the availability of gas chromatograph mass spectrometry (GCMS) to measure THC content and pharmacokinetic smoking machines to determine the amount consumed. The smoking machines would need to be calibrated to the consumption mode and a user's unique style of inhalation. This protocol lies well beyond the mechanics and budget of most field work.

On the other hand, this chapter has provided techniques for approximating the THC consumption in a cannabis use session that are inexpensive and appropriate to field research and, if refined, potentially for medical treatment. These procedures identify the questions to be asked, the language to be used, and the calculations to be performed based on the data obtained regarding the names, costs, and perceived quality of the cannabis being consumed.

Beyond question design, the pilot studies indicate that modestly-priced, convenient scientific equipment can be used effectively in the field. In the hands of an informed field researcher, digital scales and hand-held microscopes can provide reasonable estimates of cannabis quantity and quality.. Most importantly, field researchers can train study subjects on site to use the tools so that the researchers can avoid handling illegal substances. Gaining subject cooperation can be straightforward. In our experience, many cannabis users appreciate the opportunity to learn more about the quantity and quality of their cannabis. We found that even long-standing daily users often did not possess good estimates of how much a joint or a single hit of cannabis weighs and actually costs them. Despite a self-reported 10-a-day blunt habit, the experienced dealer who participated in the measurement experiments reported he could not estimate the number of hits in a blunt. Furthermore, his clients were shocked to learn that each hit from a blunt of 700mg of high-quality cannabis cost $0.40 or more, at the dealer's friends' prices—to them an exorbitantly high cost per hit.

Whether users outside of clinical settings are predisposed toward higher degrees of intoxication based on their consumption of higher potency cannabis—and whether that results in higher likelihood of dependence—are questions, however, that can only be addressed through greater methodological attention to smoking intensity and its quantification in the future. It is the unequivocal finding of this chapter that training field researchers to be sensitive to the multiple ways in which cannabis is consumed, cultivated, and marketed is an important step in that direction.

Acknowledgments

Preparation of this chapter was supported by a grant from the National Institute on Drug Abuse (1RO1 DA/CA 13690-05), and by the Behavioral Science Training in Drug Abuse Research program sponsored by Medical and Health Association of New York City, Inc. (MHRA) and the National Development and Research Institutes (NDRI) with funding from the National Institute on Drug Abuse (5T32 DA07233-24). Points of view, opinions, and conclusions in this chapter do not necessarily represent the official position of the U.S. Government, MHRA, or NDRI. The authors gratefully acknowledge the contributions of Gregory Falkin and project ethnographers, Flutura Bardhi, Doris Randolph, and Anthony Nguyen. Most importantly, however, we would like to acknowledge the contributions of Dr. Bruce D. Johnson to this chapter. He was involved with all aspects of this study until his unexpected passing in February, 2009.

References

Blair, E., Sudman, S., Bradburn, N., & Stocking, C. (1977). How to ask questions about drinking and sex: Response effects in measuring consumer behavior. *Journal of Marketing Research, 14*(3), 316-321.

Bradburn, N., Sudman, S., & Wansink, B. (2004). *Asking questions: the definitive guide to questionnaire design: for market research, political polls, and social and health questionnaires*: Jossey-Bass Inc Pub.

Cervantes, J. (2002). *Indoor marijuana horticulture*: Van Patten Pub.

Compton, W., Grant, B., Colliver, J., Glantz, M., & Stinson, F. (2004). Prevalence of marijuana use disorders in the United States: 1991-1992 and 2001-2002. *Jama, 291*(17), 2114.

Dunlap, E., Johnson, B. D., Sifaneck, S. J., & Benoit, E. (2005). Sessions, Cyphers, and Parties: Settings for Informal Social Controls of Blunt Smoking. *Journal of Ethnicity and Substance Abuse, 3/4*(43-77).

EMCDDA. (2004). European Monitoring Centre for Drugs and Drug Addiction. EMCDDA Insights: An overview of cannabis potency in

Europe. Office for Official Publications of the European Communities, Belgium.

Gieringer, D. (1999). Medical cannabis potency testing project. *Multidisciplinary Association for Psychedelic Studies Newsletter, 9*(3), 20-22.

Golub, A., Bruce D. Johnson, Eloise Dunlap. (2005). The Growth in Marijuana Use Among American Youths in the 1990s and The Extent of Blunts Smoking. *Journal of Ethnicity and Substance Abuse, 3/4*, 1-21.

Grotenhermen, F. (2003). Pharmacokinetics and pharmacodynamics of cannabinoids. *Clinical pharmacokinetics, 42*(4), 327-360.

Harrison, L., Erickson, P., Korf, D., Brochu, S., & Benschop, A. (2007). How much for a dime bag? An exploration of youth drug markets. *Drug and Alcohol Dependence, 90*, S27-S39.

Hazekamp, A., Ruhaak, R., Zuurman, L., van Gerven, J., & Verpoorte, R. (2006). Evaluation of a vaporizing device (Volcano®) for the pulmonary administration of tetrahydrocannabinol. *Journal of pharmaceutical sciences, 95*(6), 1308-1317.

Herning, R., Hooker, W., & Jones, R. (1986). Tetrahydrocannabinol content and differences in marijuana smoking behavior. *Psychopharmacology, 90*(2), 160-162.

Hurley, J., West, J., & Ehleringer, J. (2010). Tracing retail cannabis in the United States: Geographic origin and cultivation patterns. *International Journal of Drug Policy, 21*(3), 222-228.

Johnson, B. D., Bardhi, F., Sifaneck, S. J., & Dunlap, E. (2005). Marijuana Argot as Subculture Threads: Social Constructions by Users in New York City. *British Journal of Criminology, 46*(1), 46-77.

Johnson, B. D., & Golub, A. (2007). The potential for accurately measuring behavioral and economic dimensions of consumption, prices, and markets for illegal drugs. *Drug and Alcohol Dependence, 90*(S), S16-S26.

Midanik, L. (1994). Comparing usual quantity/frequency and graduated frequency scales to assess yearly alcohol consumption: results from the 1990 US National Alcohol Survey. *Addiction, 89*(4), 407-412.

Midanik, L., & Hines, A. (1991). 'Unstandard' ways of answering standard questions: protocol analysis in alcohol survey research. *Drug and Alcohol Dependence, 27*(3), 245-252.

NESARC. (2006). Alcohol Use and Alcohol Use Disorders in the United States: Main Findings from the 2001-2002 National Epidemiologic Survey on Alcohol and Related Conditions. Alcohol Epidemiologic Data Reference Manual 8(1). NIH Publications No. 05-5737.

NLAES. (2002). Alcohol Consumption and Problems in the General Population: Findings From the 1992 National Longitudinal Alcohol Epidemiologic Survey, NIH Publication No. 02-4997

NRC. (2001). Consumption data. In: Manski, C.F., Pepper, J.V., Petrie, C.V. (Eds.), Informing America's Policy on Illegal Drugs: What We Don't Know Keeps Hurting Us. National Research Council /National Academy Press, Washington, DC.

Perez-Reyes, M., Di Guiseppi, S., Davis, K., Schindler, V., & Cook, C. (1982). Comparison of effects of marihuana cigarettes of three different potencies. *Clinical Pharmacology & Therapeutics, 31*(5), 617-624.

Ramaekers, J., Moeller, M., Van Ruitenbeek, P., Theunissen, E., Schneider, E., & Kauert, G. (2006). Cognition and motor control as a function of [Delta] 9-THC concentration in serum and oral fluid: limits of impairment. *Drug and Alcohol Dependence, 85*(2), 114-122.

Rosenthal, E., Newhart, S., 2004. The big book of buds. Vol. 2 : More Marijuana Varieties from the World's Great Seed Breeders. Quick American Archives, Oakland, Calif.

Rosenthal, E., Newhart, S., 2001. The Big Book of Buds: Marijuana Varieties from the World's Great Seed Breeders. Quick American Archives, Oakland, Calif.

Ream, G., Benoit, E., Johnson, B., & Dunlap, E. (2008). Smoking tobacco along with marijuana increases symptoms of cannabis dependence. *Drug and Alcohol Dependence, 95*(3), 199.

Sifaneck, S., Kaplan, C., Dunlap, E., & Johnson, B. (2003). Blunts and blowtjes: Cannabis use practices in two cultural settings and their implications for secondary prevention. *Free Inquiry in Creative Sociology, 31*(1), 3-14.

Sifaneck, S. J., Ream, G., Johnson, B. D., & Dunlap, E. (2007). Retail Marijuana Purchases in Designer and Commercial Markets in New York City: Sales Units, Weights, and Prices per Gram. *Drug and Alcohol Dependence, 90S*, S40-51.

Single, E., & Wortley, S. (1994). A comparison of alternative measures of alcohol consumption in the Canadian National Survey of alcohol and drug use. *Addiction, 89*(4), 395-399.

Strunin, L. (2001). Assessing alcohol consumption: developments from qualitative research methods. *Social Science & Medicine, 53*(2), 215-226.

Walters, J. (2002, Sept. 1). Pot Use in America / CON / Marijuana today: Setting the record straight, Editorial, *San Francisco Chronicle*. Retrieved from http://articles.sfgate.com/2002-09-01/opinion/17560932_1_today-s-marijuana-thc-sinsemilla. Last accessed 7-14-2010.

In: Marijuana: Uses, Effects and the Law
Editor: Andrea S. Rojas
ISBN 978-1-61209-206-5

Chapter 3

PUBLIC HEALTH PERSPECTIVES ON THE MEDICAL USE OF CANNABIS: THE INFLUENCE OF CANNABIS LEGISLATION ON VULNERABLE POPULATIONS

David S. Black*[*], *Leyla Irzabayova, N. Ryan Rysyk and Steve Sussman

Institute for Health Promotion & Disease Prevention Research, University of Southern California, Keck School of Medicine, Alhambra, CA, USA

ABSTRACT

Cannabis remains an illegal substance according to the U.S. Federal Government despite some recent research suggesting that medical cannabis use is safe and has therapeutic potential for some vulnerable populations with chronic medical conditions. A public health perspective suggests that such legislation leads to increased health risks to vulnerable populations and

[*] Please address all correspondence and reprint requests to: David S. Black, M.P.H. Institute for Health Promotion & Disease Prevention Research; University of Southern California; 1000 S. Fremont Avenue, Unit #8, Building A-5; Alhambra, CA 91803-4737. E-mail: davidbla@usc.edu

potential reductions in quality of life. The APHA was one of the first American public health associations to formally recommend cannabis as an avenue for use in medical treatment and research. The following chapter discusses some of the main issues surrounding medical cannabis use among vulnerable populations from a public health perspective. A public health perspective suggests how such legislation may result to further increase disadvantage and health problems among vulnerable populations who are in need of alternative drug therapies. It is possible that legalizing medical cannabis has greater potential benefits than harms to vulnerable populations in the medical context who are not responding well to conventional treatment. However, realistic cautions should be taken to reduce cannabis dependence, potential respiratory problems, potential for accidents, or other undesired effects, and relatively safe means for cannabis intake should continued to be explored.

The *cannabis sativa* plant, more commonly known as cannabis or marijuana, has been used medicinally for millennia and continues to play a significant role in medical treatment today. The cannabis plant provides both psychoactive and non-psychoactive medicinal products. A psychoactive substance is as a chemical agent that crosses the blood-brain barrier and alters brain function, resulting in changes in perception, cognition, mood and behavior. Psychoactive substances are typically regulated by government jurisdiction such as the Federal Government and the Food and Drug Administration (FDA) in the United States as they have the potential for abuse and dependence. Non-psychoactive cannabis-derived products have less oversight from the government and include such products as hemp oils, hemp seeds, and hemp protein. These non-psychoactive products are considered to have diuretic, anti-emetic, anti-inflammatory, anti-microbial, dietary supplement, as well as other medicinal properties (Aggarwal et al., 2009; Leizer, Ribnicky, Poulev, Dushenkov & Raskin, 2000; Lozano, 2001).

The psychoactive properties of cannabis result from various cannabinoids, which are the chemical compounds found within the dried flowers and leaves of the cannabis plant. The most well-known psychoactive cannabinoid contained within the cannabis plant is Tetrahydrocannabinol (Delta 9-THC), or THC for short. Interestingly, THC is believed to be used by the cannabis plant for self-defense against herbivores and protection from UV radiation exposure (Lydon, Teramura & Coffman, 1987; Pate, 1994). THC is most concentrated in the mature female plant's unseeded flowers and least concentrated in the leaves, stem and seeds. At least 66 cannabinoids have been isolated from the cannabis plant, but other than THC, Cannabidiol (CBD), Cannabinol (CBN)

of value will help. "Once they realize they are receiving a positive ticket for doing something good, it seems then that they calm right down and then they are appreciative," PC Rob Lindsay tells CBC. "Hopefully it will give them a chance to come be more approachable to us, communicate with us and talk to us as well down the road." And with such appealing prizes on offer, the city's young people "may start seeking out police officers in hopes of getting caught," the CBC report says.

Use #NewsfromElsewhere to stay up-to-date with our reports via Twitter.

More videos from the BBC

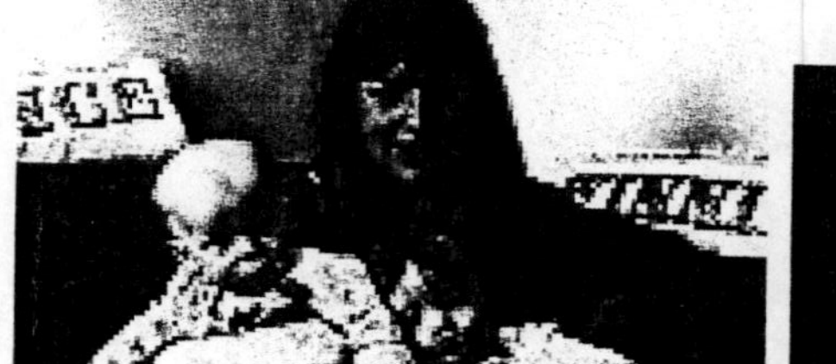

'Why I needed Danish sperm donor'

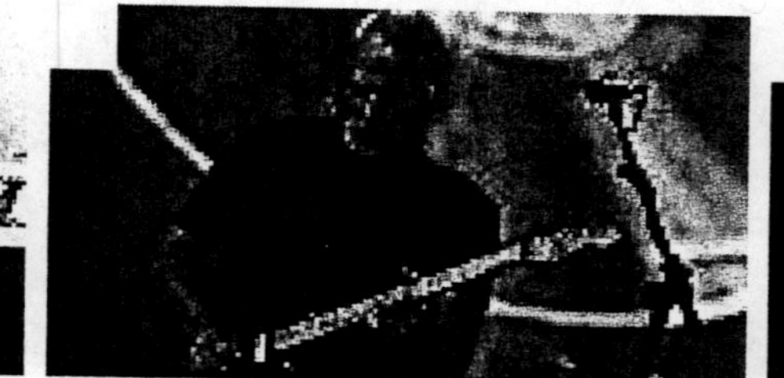

Pink Floyd 'surprised' by album response

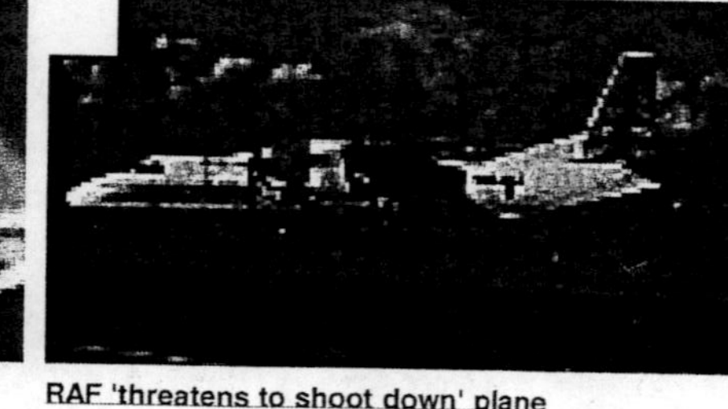

RAF 'threatens to shoot down' plane

BBC NEWS

NEWS FROM ELSEWHERE

11 November 2014 Last updated at 09:38 ET

Canada: Police force hands out 'positive tickets'

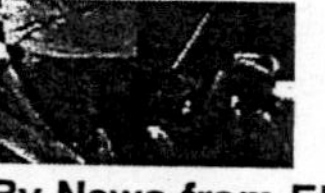

By News from Elsewhere...
...media reports from around the world, found by BBC Monitoring

A police force in Canada has started handing out rewards to young people who do good things for their community.

Officers in the city of Prince Albert, in the central province of Saskatchewan, will dish out the "positive tickets" to youngsters who are seen crossing the road safely or picking up litter, the CBC news website reports. The rewards on offer include free hamburgers, cinema tickets or a chance to see the local hockey team in action, all of which have been donated by local businesses. The initiative rewards young people who make "healthy, positive choices in relation to their behaviour, decisions or actions", the force says on its website. "One officer is recognising a group of school children that call themselves peacekeepers," Sgt Brandon ... BBC. "They have taken a peacekeeping course through the school and ... safe from bullying type situati..."

are the most prevalent natural cannabinoids and have received the most scientific attention.

The psychoactive effects of cannabinoids can be obtained through inhaled cannabis smoke and vaporized gas or through consumption of appropriately prepared baked goods or drinks which contains cannabis. The psychoactive effects of cannabis are diverse and typically differ by amount of dosage. For example, lower doses of cannabis typically produce mild sedative-hypnotic effects, whereas higher doses may also produce hallucinations, intensified emotional responses, euphoria, hallucinations, and heightened sensations. Despite the controversial psychoactive effects derived from cannabis use, cannabinoids are considered to have beneficial effects on a variety of health conditions (Costa, 2007). For example, THC is somewhat effective in improving a wide variety of medical ailments such as pain, nausea and vomiting, loss of appetite, glaucoma, spasticity, and anxiety (Watson, Benson Jr & Joy, 2000). These conditions are also increasingly being treated with cannabis-derived synthetic dronabinol and nabilone, and a combination of synthetic THC and synthesized cannabidiol.

Although a growing area of research suggests that cannabinoids can contribute to effective treatment of various ailments in the medical context, cannabis use also has specific dangers (e.g. see Sussman et al., 1996). For example, a relatively small percentage of long-term cannabis users can develop drug tolerance and dependence, and the inhalation of cannabis smoke can have a negative impact on respiratory tract health (Watson et al., 2000). Of the multiple uses of cannabis products, one of the most salient issues of ongoing debate concerns the use of cannabis to treat health conditions in the medical context. Today, local, state, and federal governments continue to disagree about medical cannabis use legislation. Cannabis use is currently prohibited by the United States Federal Government, meaning that the substance is illegal and cannabis possession and distribution are both federal offenses. However, legal medical cannabis use, which allows people to obtain and use cannabis to treat a medical condition with oversight from a health care professional without fear of legal repercussions, differs across state borders. For example, in 1996, California voters passed Proposition 215, making it the first state to allow for the medical use of cannabis. To date, there are a total of fourteen states that have passed laws eliminating criminal penalties for using cannabis for medical purposes, and at least twelve other states are considering similar legislation. The states allowing for legal medical cannabis use include California, Alaska, Oregon, Washington, Maine, Hawaii, Colorado, Nevada, Vermont, Montana, Rhode Island, New Mexico, Michigan, and New Jersey. In the vast majority of states, medical cannabis remains a criminal offense punishable by fine, time in jail, or both.

A BRIEF OVERVIEW OF THE MEDICAL USE OF CANNABIS IN THE UNITED STATES

Between 1840 and 1900, European and American medical journals published more than 100 articles on the therapeutic use of cannabis (see Grinspoon & Bakalar, 1995). During this period, cannabis was recommended for a variety of purposes such as an appetite stimulant, muscle relaxant, analgesic, hypnotic, and anticonvulsant. However, the scientific exploration of cannabis use in medical treatment began to decline in the early 20th century. This decline was mostly due to the development of alternative medications such as opiates, barbiturates, and aspirin and because the potency of cannabis was variable making dosage criteria unclear. In addition, the Marihuana Tax Act was initialized in 1937, which was the first legislation to criminalize cannabis in the United States. This legislation played a major role in reducing the medical use of cannabis as it held physicians and patients legally accountable for prescription and possession of cannabis. Public awareness of arrests for cannabis possession and distribution that resulted from this law also dissuaded physicians from prescribing medical cannabis to patients. This law also restricted access to cannabis for medical purposes. Cannabis was soon removed from the American pharmacopeia, a comprehensive reference of pharmaceutical drugs published by the medical authority, in 1944 due to political pressure to ban its use in the United States (Bonnie & Whitebread, 1974; Walsh, Nelson & Mahmoud, 2003). Although cannabis has not been placed back in the American pharmacopoeia since that time, in 1986 the Food and Drug Administration authorized the use of its active element, THC, for medical purposes such as treating nausea and vomiting side effects in patients receiving chemotherapy (Walsh et al., 2003).

Presently in the United States, cannabis is classified as a Schedule I drug under the Controlled Substances Act (CSA). This scheduling characterizes cannabis as having high potential for abuse, contends that cannabis lacks an accepted medical use, and specifies that it is unsafe for use even under medical supervision. This scheduling represents the United States Federal Government's fight against the abuse of drugs and other substances. It has been well-argued that the prohibition of medical marijuana is based on political ideology and not the accumulated scientific evidence (see Carter & Mirken, 2006). Further, the beneficial effects of cannabis noted in scientific reports and by public health officials contradict these notions that cannabis lacks an accepted medical use and that it is unsafe under the guidance of medical supervision. Consequently, at the close of the first decade of the 21st century, interest in the medical use of cannabis is burgeoning once again, and scientific evidence is continuing to accumulate in some states regarding the potential of cannabis as an effective therapy for certain medical conditions. Therefore, as state and local governments begin to re-evaluate the therapeutic effects of cannabis, it is important to consider the impact of medical cannabis legislation on specific populations who are most influenced by such legislation.

The following section discusses some of the main issues surrounding medical cannabis use among vulnerable populations from a public health perspective. This is an important perspective given that a very broad oversight of population health is directed by the field of public health. Examining the public health perspective is useful in that it provides an understanding of how vulnerable populations are affected by cannabis legislation. Moreover, a public health perspective suggests how such legislation may result to further increase disadvantage and health problems among vulnerable populations who are in need of alternative drug therapies such as cannabis.

PUBLIC HEALTH AND MEDICAL CANNABIS USE

Public health is both an empirical and applied field of science that aims to prevent disease and promote health and wellbeing among general and vulnerable populations. Some main objectives of public health include: (1) assessing and monitoring the health of populations to identify health problems, (2) formulating and influencing public policies designed to solve the identified health problems, and (3) assuring that populations have proper access to appropriate and cost-effective care (MedicineNet, 2010). Cannabis use is relevant to all three goals of public health, such that the field of public health is then concerned with: (1) monitoring cannabis use/ abuse to determine the frequency and impact of cannabis on the general population and within vulnerable subgroups, (2) influencing policy to allow access to medical cannabis where cannabis is shown to be effective, and (3) evaluating the efficacy of cannabis use as an effective medical treatment while assuring access to those vulnerable populations that will benefit from cannabis. As such, the field of public health has an important role to play in cannabis policy, and has influence such policy for over a decade.

The American Public Health Association (APHA) is the oldest and largest organization of health care professionals in the world. It was also the first American public health organization to recommend clinical research on cannabis and the use of cannabis in the context of medical treatment (American Public Health Association, 1995). The APHA has played a significant role in the more recent history of medical cannabis legislation. The 1995 APHA endorsement of cannabis was based on the rationale that greater harm to population health is caused by legal consequences of cannabis prohibition than possible risks of medical use. The APHA called for reform by encouraging that further research be conducted to determine the medical benefits of cannabis. The APHA specifically encouraged research on the therapeutic properties of various cannabinoids contained within cannabis, and research on alternative methods of administration to decrease smoking-related harm. In addition, the APHA urged legislation change to make cannabis available as a legal medicine where shown safe and effective and to allow access to therapeutic cannabis through the Investigational New Drug Program. Although legislation to allow access to medical marijuana continues to change at a slow pace in the United States, there is promising evidence that the recommendations made by the APHA are materializing to further support medical cannabis legislation reform.

The field of public health continues to play a major role in overseeing the medical delivery of cannabis today. For example, the California Department of Public Health administers the Medical Marijuana Identification Card (MMIC) program and oversees the Medical Marijuana Program (MMP), organizations which allow access to medical cannabis for patients residing in California. Services include the provision of a medical marijuana identification card and placement within a patient registry program for qualified patients and their caregivers. This registry system allows law enforcement and the public to verify the validity of qualified patient or caregiver's legal authorization to administer, possess, grow, transport and use medical cannabis in California. To facilitate the verification of authorized cardholders, the cannabis registry is available on the internet. Upon obtaining a recommendation from their physician for use of medicinal cannabis, patients and their primary caregivers may apply for, and be issued, a Medical Marijuana Identification Card. Since the inception of the program in 2004, there have been over 42,500 cards issued in California (California Department of Public Health, 2010), indicating a growing need for access to medical cannabis in states where medical cannabis is legal. It is important to note that this need for cannabis access may partially be represented by an increase in individuals abusing these privileges to gain access to cannabis for recreational use.

THE BENEFITS OF MEDICAL CANNABIS USE FROM A PUBLIC HEALTH PERSPECTIVE

A main public health objective is to assure that the most beneficial medical care be offered to vulnerable populations in order to reduce disadvantage and promote wellbeing. A vulnerable population in the medical context can be defined as a group that suffers from chronic conditions such as cancer, HIV/AIDS, diabetes mellitus, Inflammatory Bowel Disease (IBD), Crohn's Disease, rheumatoid arthritis, multiple sclerosis as well as other conditions, and that is not responding completely to conventional medical treatment. Possibly, these populations may benefit from the effects of cannabis use beyond the effects obtained by conventional drugs. However, due to its problems with legality, medical cannabis use is an understudied agent for treating symptoms resulting from these chronic conditions.

Symptoms resulting from chronic conditions may include pain, psychological distress, loss of appetite, weight loss, and other ailments. Moreover, antiretroviral and chemotherapy treatments often result in unintended side-effects that cause discomfort such as nausea and vomiting. Up to 75 percent of chronic disease patients experience nausea and vomiting side-effects from treatment, and patients report these symptoms as highly stressful events that negatively impact their quality of life (Schwartzberg, 2007). These distressing side effects can lead to depression, anxiety and a feeling of helplessness (Wilcox, Fetting, Nettesheim & Abeloff, 1982), all of which are psychosocial ailments associated with poorer treatment outcomes. The legalization of medical cannabis in some states has allowed for the scientific investigation of cannabis in these regions, and studies have yielded promising results for the therapeutic value of cannabis as a treatment for several health conditions.

Recent scientific evidence gives some support for the efficacy of cannabis as an adjunct treatment to ease many symptoms of chronic conditions. For example, as compared to conventional drugs and placebo, the antiemetic (i.e., medications used to prevent vomiting) efficacy of cannabis and its cannabinoid derivatives appears to be as good or slightly better in symptom reduction among cancer patients receiving chemotherapy (Rocha, Stefano, Haiek, Oliveria & Da Silveira, 2008). These results show that cannabinoids have some proven effectiveness for anti-emetic use. The cannabinoid receptors, located in areas of the brainstem that control emesis, are thought to play a key role in this mechanism (Martin & Wiley, 2004). In addition, some patients actually prefer cannabis use over conventional drugs, indicating that cannabis may impose less unwanted side-effects on some patients as compared to conventional drugs. The variety of options for cannabis delivery to the body is also important especially when considering that antiemetic pills are often an ineffective method to administer in patients already experiencing severe nausea or vomiting because of difficulty swallowing. Thus, the inhalation of cannabis offers a better method of administration for patients by means of its ease of use and rapidity of onset.

Some studies suggest that cannabis may be a useful treatment for people with advanced stages of chronic disease, which is a period of disease that often does not respond well to conventional drug treatment. For example, advanced stages of cancer, HIV/AIDS, diabetes, fibromyalgia, and multiple sclerosis impose symptoms such as cachexia and/or neuropathic pain (i.e., chronic pain caused by tissue and nerve damage). Cachexia is loss of weight, muscle atrophy, fatigue, and significant loss of appetite in patients with chronic disease who are not actively trying to lose weight. Cachexia signifies that an underlying chronic disease has progressed and is likely to cause mortality. Patient response to standard treatment at this stage is typically poor, and patients seek to maintain a quality of life with the least amount of pain and treatment side-effects as possible. The most promising treatment is to deliver drugs that reduce pain and increase patient appetite in order to reduce or reverse weight loss. Cannabis has long been used by HIV-infected patients as an appetite enhancer and pain-relieving medication (Furler, Einarson, Millson, Walmsley & Bendayan, 2004). Also, its ability to reduce nausea is one promising method for treating cachexia in patients with advanced chronic disease (Martin & Wiley, 2004). Although other medications may be more effective than cannabis for symptoms of chronic disease problems, they are not equally effective for all patients. In this respect, cannabis is an important agent to treat subgroups of patients who do not react to conventional medications and need alternative agents to treat their chronic symptoms.

Chronic pain is often a symptom encountered by chronic disease patients. Pain symptoms are often difficult to treat with conventional drugs without the imposition of substantial negative side-effects. Moreover, drug interactions between pain medications and antiretroviral/ cancer medications often result in unwanted symptoms. For example, neuropathic pain impacts a substantial percentage of chronic disease patients, and these pain symptoms can be modulated by cannabis use. This is not surprising considering that cannabinoids have been used as analgesics for more than 3000 years (Mechoulam & Ben-Shabat, 1999). There is a convincing line of research that supports the use of cannabis to treat pain symptoms in some patients.

A prospective randomized placebo-controlled trial conducted with HIV-positive hospital inpatients showed that smoked cannabis was well tolerated, within an acceptable safety margin, and effectively relieved chronic neuropathic pain (Abrams et al., 2007). These positive results were replicated in a Phase II, double-blind, placebo-controlled trial among HIV-positive patients with neuropathic pain (Ellis et al., 2008), which suggested that the pain relieving benefits of cannabis use are comparable to conventional oral drugs used for chronic neuropathic pain. A consecutive series of randomized, double-blind, placebo-controlled, single-patient, crossover trials among patients with multiple sclerosis, spinal cord injury, brachial plexus damage, and limb amputation concluded that cannabis medicinal extracts can improve neurogenic symptoms unresponsive to standard treatments, with predictable moderate side-effects and good tolerability (Wade, Robson, House, Makela & Aram, 2003). A host of other studies have supported the effectiveness of cannabis as a treatment for chronic pain, and reviews of this literature have suggested cannabis is one effective agent for medical use among some patients with chronic diseases (Cinti, 2009; Corless et al., 2009).

Debilitating chronic pain occurs in 50–70% of multiple sclerosis patients. A review of randomized, double-blinded placebo-controlled trials of cannabinoid-based treatments for multiple sclerosis-related neuropathic pain in adults indicated that cannabinoids including the cannabidiol THC spray were effective in treating neuropathic pain in multiple sclerosis (Iskedjian, Bereza, Gordon, Piwko & Einarson, 2006). In addition, a randomized, double-blind, placebo-controlled, parallel-group trial found that cannabis use reduced pain and sleep disturbance among patients with multiple sclerosis (Rog, Nurmikko, Friede & Young, 2005). Furthermore, a line of empirical evidence suggests that spasticity, an involuntary increase in muscle tone or rapid muscle contractions that is highly distressing to multiple sclerosis patients, can be attenuated to some degree through clinician-monitored cannabis treatment (Lakhan & Rowland, 2009).

Cannabis use for other chronic diseases has been understudied and much less is known about the therapeutic efficacy of cannabis in these contexts. Some initial research and anecdotal evidence suggests that cannabis may also be useful as a treatment adjunct for glaucoma (Tomida et al., 2006), as an antiepileptic (Mortati, 2007), as a treatment neurodegenerative disorders (Luvone, Esposito, De Filippis, Scuderi & Steardo, 2009) and other conditions. Because the evidence for medical cannabis use for these conditions has been scant and contradictory, further research is needed in these areas to determine if cannabis and its derivatives are useful for patients with these medical conditions as well as others. Although the benefits of cannabis use among vulnerable populations living with chronic diseases are evident in the scientific literature, a public health perspective also takes caution to note the potential concerns of medical cannabis use.

Public Health Concerns regarding Medical Cannabis Use

Cannabis is not an efficacious treatment for all patients with chronic conditions. Thus, there are several public health concerns previously noted regarding cannabis use in the medical context (Sussman et al., 1996). For example, there are undesired short-term side effects of cannabis use encountered by some patients that must be carefully monitored by clinicians when delivered as medical treatment. Commonly observed adverse effects associated with the use of cannabis agents include drowsiness, dizziness, speech impediments, memory impairment and confusion (Turcotte et al., 2010). Many of these side effects are characterized as non-serious ailments, and are dependent on the individual patient, including their symptomatic profile, concomitant illnesses and previous medications and therapy. Thus, care must be given by physicians prescribing cannabis to patients who may be sensitive to the adverse side-effects of cannabis use. In addition, there is some anecdotal evidence and case studies that have also suggested that cannabis use may be associated with psychiatric disorders, especially among previously high-risk patients (Pierre, 2010).

Second, there are longer-term more serious consequences of cannabis use to consider. Cannabis smoking as well as any other type of smoking, such as tobacco use, is associated with abnormalities of cells lining the human respiratory tract due to carcinogens and tars inhaled during smoking (Sussman et al., 1996). Thus, it is not surprising that cannabis smoking has been linked with sensitivity to respiratory illness, cancer, impaired respiratory function, and lung damage in some studies (Aldington et al., 2007; Tashkin, 1999). In addition, cannabis-dependent respondents report higher rates of wheezing, shortness of breath, chest tightness and morning sputum production after controlling for the effects of tobacco use (Taylor et al., 2002). However, there is conflicting evidence which suggests cannabis smoking is not associated with several of these ailments (Llewellyn, Linklater, Bell, Johnson & Warnakulasuriya, 2004; Rosenblatt, Daling, Chen, Sherman & Schwartz, 2004; Sidney, Quesenberry Jr, Friedman & Tekawa, 1997), particularly if not heavily smoked or used with vaporizers (Van Dam & Earleywine, 2010) or inhalers (e.g., Sativex; Guy and Stott, 2005). At least one population-based study failed to identify any significant positive association between cannabis smoking and the occurrence of head, neck and lung cancers, whereas tobacco smoking was a major risk factor for these conditions (Hashibe et al., 2006). Confirmative studies are needed to determine the causal relationships between cannabis smoking and these long-term ailments. Until these studies provide confirmatory evidence, it is best that cannabis products be delivered in a non-smoked form to clinical populations, when possible, to assure safety. Alternative cannabis administration techniques include vaporized cannabis and buccal sprays. Studies show that these techniques are safer and are associated with decreased respiratory problems as compared with smoked cannabis (Earleywine & Barnwell, 2007).

Long-term concerns regarding cannabis use also pertain to patient abuse of cannabis and the development of cannabis dependence resulting from heavy chronic use of cannabis. Symptoms such as loss of control over cannabis use and cannabis withdrawal are indications of substance abuse and dependence and may require treatment for successful cessation (Budney et al., 2003; Budney, Novey and Hughes, 1999; Stephens, Roffman & Simpson, 1993). Substance abuse and dependence have significant negative personal, social, and medical consequences, and these consequences are of main interest to public health, thus medical cannabis use must be prescribed only during the course of required treatment and carefully monitored. When patients become dependent on cannabis and attempt cessation, they may encounter withdrawal symptoms such as restlessness, irritability, mild agitation, insomnia, sleep disturbance, nausea, and cramping. Cannabis withdrawal is relatively short-lived after cessation compared to other legal substances such as alcohol and tobacco. Still, as with other substances, up to 70% of marijuana addicts may relapse within a year of trying to quit (Sussman et al., 1996).

As with other drugs, cannabis users can develop dependence, however, cannabis dependence is reported by a very small amoung of cannabis users. The estimated prevalence of dependence among cannabis users is about 4% in the United States general population across the lifespan (Anthony, Warner & Kessler, 1994). This is in relation to a 24% estimated prevalence of dependence on tobacco and 14% prevalence of dependence on alcohol across the lifespan (Anthony, Warner & Kessler, 1994). However, other studies have reported that more people abuse cannabis than other illicit drugs (Sussman et al., in press). However, little is known about prevalence estimates of dependence with specific reference to medical cannabis use, which is a type of use presumed to be less related to dependency considering that cannabis use is under physician supervision. Moreover, the general populations use of cannabis is often confounded by multiple drug use and psychopathology (Stephens et al., 1993), making cannabis dependence prevalence estimates in the general population an overestimate of cannabis-specific dependence.

Present data on drug use progression neither support nor refute the suggestion that cannabinoid availability as medicine would increase cannabis abuse and dependence in the medical context. Most importantly, this question is beyond the issues normally considered for the medical use of drugs. In general, existing findings are consistent with the notion that cannabis use has relatively low potential for abuse when closely monitored as compared to other medications with abuse potential. Moreover, medical cannabis use is very rare by comparison with non-medical use, and is often only used for a short-term period comprising the extent of medical treatment (e.g., during chemotherapy treatment; Hall and Degenhardt, 2010). Moreover, medical cannabis used does not appear to compromise other substance abuse treatment outcomes in patients enrolled in substance abuse programs (Ronald, 2010).

Third, public health is also concerned with indirect influences of medical cannabis use on the general population's health. Patients who use medical cannabis also drive motor vehicles and have vocations that require using machinery. Some evidence suggests that cannabis is linked with motor vehicle accidents, which is a major area of public health supervision. Cannabis use effects motor coordination, attention, and decision-making; all of these cognitive factor are important when driving. Meta-analyses have concluded that cannabis use generally slows driver performance and may increase distractability, particularly in complex driving situations (Anderson et al., 2010; Laberge & Ward, 2004; Ramaekers, Berghaus, van Laar & Drummer, 2004). However, it is unclear whether this association found in previous literature is confounded by other drug use such as alcohol and illicit drugs. For example, toxicology assays indicated that cannabis use by itself was not associated with car crashes among drivers presenting to an emergency room in one study (Lowenstein & Koziol-McLain, 2001), but not others (Brookoff et al., 1994). Moreover, cannabis use did not significantly impair driving performance in two simulated driving performance studies (Liguori, Gatto & Jarrett, 2002; Liguori, Gatto, Jarrett, Vaughn McCall & Brown, 2003). Therefore, it has been suggested that an increased risk of accidents among cannabis users is more related to personal characteristics rather than the effects of cannabis itself (Fergusson & Horwood, 2001).

Overall, any impairing effects of cannabis use appear to be less severe than those of alcohol, but the collected evidence has led to the recommendation to avoid driving while under the influence of cannabis (Liguori, 2007). The risk of traffic accidents by the medical use of medication can be remediated as with any other prescribed medication that affects perception and motor coordination. To address this issue, labels on cannabis prescriptions should inform patients to not drive under the influence of their medication, and this labeling practice should be carefully regulated by medical authorities. In summary, it is evident that patients should not operate dangerous machinery or drive cars while under the influence of cannabis, as with most other psychoactive prescriptions.

Finally, cannabis may socially stigmatize vulnerable populations due to criminal prosecution of medical marijuana users. Vulnerable populations use medical cannabis to treat their medical conditions under the threat they will be prosecuted for possessing cannabis. This social stigma often leads to incorrectly labeling medical cannabis users as deviant or as drug abusers. Criminal prosecution in this manner has long-lasting effects on the cannabis user, their family, and the broader social context, which are all health issues under the supervision of public health. The actual and perceived stigma resulting from criminalizing cannabis also dissuades some patients from using cannabis as a treatment option even though this treatment may be of benefit to them.

Criminalizing medical cannabis also creates public health problems with safe access to cannabis. Patients who seek medical cannabis but do not have legal access to safe dispensaries have to illegally pursue cannabis. This creates high-risk situations for the patient as they become involved in illegal drug dealing, which often involves gang-related activity, exposure to illicit drugs, unregulated contents (i.e., laced cannabis), and violence. Proponets of public health recommends that vulnerable populations should have safe access to effective medical treatment, and therefore are against criminalizing those patients who seek out cannabis as a therapeutic treatment. Of course, there also is the possibility that recent proliferation of medical cannabis clinics throughout California have resulted in an increase in fallacious cannabis prescriptions for recreational use. Thus, ongoing monitoring at the government level is needed to regulate these clinics in order to assure appropriate prescribing and dispensing of medical cannabis to prevent unregulated recreational use in the general population.

CONCLUSIONS REGARDING MEDICAL CANNABIS FROM A PUBLIC HEALTH PERSPECTIVE

Medical cannabis remains an illegal substance according to the United States Federal Government and to the vast majority of states, despite some recent research suggesting that medical cannabis use is safe and has therapeutic potential for some vulnerable populations with chronic medical conditions. The Federal Controlled Substances Act classifies cannabis as a Schedule I drug, which is a scheduling that denotes cannabis as an agent that has no accepted medical utility and one that has a high potential for abuse. Moreover, a 2005 Supreme Court decision (*Gonzales v. Raich*) made clear that regardless of state laws, federal law enforcement has the authority to arrest and prosecute physicians who prescribe or dispense cannabis and patients who possess or cultivate cannabis. Consequently, the federal government criminalizes the acts of prescribing, dispensing, and possessing cannabis for any purpose. However, according to the established scientific evidence, this classification is scientifically groundless, and a public health perspective suggests that such legislation of medical cannabis leads to increased health risks to vulnerable populations and potential reductions in quality of life.

The APHA was one of the first American public health associations to formally recommend cannabis as an avenue for use in medical treatment and research. Similar recommendations have been endorsed by several national health organizations at some point in their history. These recommendations for the re-evaluation of cannabis as a federal Schedule I drug allows for further clinical research to test the therapeutic efficacy of cannabis to increase the health and quality of life of vulnerable medical populations. Some of the organizations that opted for reconsideration of medical cannabis use have included the Institute of Medicine, American Medical Association, American Academy of Family Physicians, American College of Physicians, American Pain Foundation, National Multiple Sclerosis Society, and American Cancer Society.

Research efforts to verify the therapeutic utility of medical cannabis and legalize its use among patients promotes access to safe and effective treatment for vulnerable populations. Currently, as a Schedule I controlled substance, research is prevented, on a large scale, from elucidating the therapeutic utility of cannabinoid-based medicines, which may advance effective care for vulnerable populations. Reconsidering current legislation in this way allows for the establishment of evidence-based practices in this area. This is important considering that scientific data indicate the potential therapeutic value of cannabinoid drugs for symptoms such as pain relief, control of nausea and vomiting, and appetite stimulation for vulnerable population with chronic conditions, which have been discussed in this chapter.

The rationale for medical cannabis use by the APHA is convincing and based in scientific evidence accumulated to date. Some key points made regarding cannabis use in the 1995 American Public Health Association's Endorsement on Medical Marijuana included (1) cannabis has a wide acute margin of safety for use under medical supervision and cannot cause lethal reactions, (2) cannabis seems to work differently from many conventional medications for several medical problems, making it a possible option for patients resistant to conventional medications, (3) patients and their families may be forced to break the law in order to obtain access to cannabis when conventional treatments are not effective, (4) current cannabis laws make criminals out of vulnerable populations, and illegal routes of accessing cannabis creates a risk for obtaining contaminated medicine, and (5) cannabis was wrongfully classified as a Schedule I drug because evidence for its therapeutic potential has been found. Thus, the APHA has adopted a resolution (7014) on Marijuana and the Law which urged federal and state drug laws to exclude cannabis from rigid classification as a narcotic.

From a public health perspective, it is possible that legalizing medical cannabis has greater potential benefits than harms to vulnerable populations in the medical context who are not responding well to conventional treatment. Thus, from a public health perspective, which is concerned with providing the most effective treatment to vulnerable populations in order to promote wellbeing, cannabis is recommended as a legal treatment option for those patients who can benefit from the effects of cannabis use. This requires legalization in order for physicians to prescribe cannabis and for patients to access and use cannabis safely and with protection from criminal stigma. Moreover, medical cannabis legalization is necessary in order for research to further examine the therapeutic properties of various cannabinoids, the methods of administration of cannabinoids to decrease the effects related to smoking, and the specific medical populations and diseases that cannabis use shows the greatest effectiveness. This does not mean that the dangers of cannabis use also should not be further investigated and made clear to patients. Realistic cautions should be taken to reduce cannabis dependence, potential respiratory problems, potential for accidents, or other undesired effects, and relatively safe means for cannabis intake should continued to be explored.

For those states currently supporting legal cannabis use and those states which are now beginning this transformation, there are important notes of caution to assure that medical cannabis use remains a recognized treatment option for vulnerable populations. First, it is important that physicians prescribing medical cannabis to patients provide full disclosures of risks and benefits necessary for informed consent to assure that patients are well-informed about the risks and benefits of cannabis use. Second, it is important that more conventional treatments be delivered to vulnerable populations prior to using cannabis; with the current evidence, cannabis should be a secondary response given to those patients who do not respond well to more conventional treatments. Third, because smoked cannabis is a crude cannabinoid delivery method that is harmful to the respiratory tract, it is recommended that cannabis be delivered by less harmful methods when feasible. Fourth, medical cannabis should be prescribed to patients with conditions for which there is reasonable expectation of efficacy, and not as a general adjunct treatment for all conditions. Finally, all cannabis treatment should be administered under medical supervision with routine assessments to screen for substance abuse and ongoing medical efficacy. Exercising caution as such is important for medical cannabis to increase in availability among vulnerable populations in order to treat their health conditions and promote wellbeing among this disadvantaged group.

REFERENCES

Abrams, D. I., Jay, C. A., Shade, S. B., Vizoso, H., Reda, H., Press, S., et al. (2007). Cannabis in painful HIV-associated sensory neuropathy: A randomized placebo-controlled trial. *Neurology*, *68*(7), 515.

Aggarwal, S. K., Carter, G. T., Sullivan, M. D., ZumBrunnen, C., Morrill, R., & Mayer, J. D. (2009). Medicinal use of cannabis in the united states: Historical perspectives, current trends, and future directions. *Journal of Opioid Management*, *5*(3), 153.

Aldington, S., Williams, M., Nowitz, M., Weatherall, M., Pritchard, A., McNaughton, A., et al. (2007). Effects of cannabis on pulmonary structure, function and symptoms. *Thorax*, *62*(12), 1058.

American Public Health Association (1995). The american public health association's endorsement on medical marijuana. 9513: Access to therapeutic marijuana/cannabis. Available from http://Www.Drugpolicy. Org/docuploads/aphaendorse.Pdf.

Anderson, B. M., Rizzo, M., Block, R. I., Pearlson, G. D., & O'Leary, D. S. (2010). Sex differences in the effects of marijuana on simulated driving performance. *Journal of Psychoactive Drugs*, *42*(1), 19.

Anthony, J. C., Warner, L. A., & Kessler, R. C. (1994). Comparative epidemiology of dependence on tobacco, alcohol, controlled substances, and inhalants: Basic findings from the national comorbidity survey. *Experimental and Clinical Psychopharmacology*, *2*(3), 244-268.

Bonnie, R. J. & Whitebread, C. H. (1974). *The marihuana conviction: A history of marihuana prohibition in the united states.* Charlottesville, VA: University Press.

Budney, A. J., Moore, B. A., Vandrey, R. G., & Hughes, J. R. (2003). The time course and significance of cannabis withdrawal. *Journal of Abnormal Psychology*, *112*(3), 393-402.

Budney, A. J., Novy, P. L., & Hughes, J. R. (1999). Marijuana withdrawal among adults seeking treatment for marijuana dependence. *Addiction*, *94*(9), 1311-1322.

California Department of Public Health (2010). Medical marijuana program (MMP) facts and figures. Prepared by the County Health Services Branch. Retrieved 08/17/2010 from http://Www.Cdph.Ca.Gov/programs/ MMP/documents/web%20fact%20sheet%206-9-10.Pdf.

Carter, G. T. & Mirken, B. (2006). Medical marijuana: Politics trumps science at the FDA. *Medgenmed*, *8*(2), 46.

Cinti, S. (2009). Medical marijuana in hiv-positive patients: What do we know? *Journal of the International Association of Physicians in AIDS Care*, *8*(6), 342.

Corless, I. B., Lindgren, T., Holzemer, W., Robinson, L., Moezzi, S., Kirksey, K., et al. (2009). Marijuana effectiveness as an HIV self-care strategy. *Clinical Nursing Research*, *18*(2), 172.

Costa, B. (2007). On the pharmacological properties of δ9-tetrahydrocannabinol (THC). *Chemistry & Biodiversity*, *4*(8), 1664-1677.

Earleywine, M. & Barnwell, S. S. (2007). Decreased respiratory symptoms in cannabis users who vaporize. *Harm Reduction Journal*, *4*(1), 11.

Ellis, R. J., Toperoff, W., Vaida, F., van den Brande, G., Gonzales, J., Gouaux, B., et al. (2008). Smoked medicinal cannabis for neuropathic pain in HIV: A randomized, crossover clinical trial. *Neuropsychopharmacology, 34*(3), 672-680.

Fergusson, D. M. & Horwood, L. J. (2001). Cannabis use and traffic accidents in a birth cohort of young adults. *Accident, Analysis and Prevention, 33*(6), 703.

Furler, M. D., Einarson, T. R., Millson, M., Walmsley, S., & Bendayan, R. (2004). Medicinal and recreational marijuana use by patients infected with HIV. *AIDS Patient Care and STDs, 18*(4), 215-228.

Grinspoon, L. & Bakalar, J. B. (1995). Marijuana as medicine-a plea for reconsideration. *JAMA, 273*(23), 1875-1876.

Guy, G. & Stott, C. (2005). The development of sativex® a natural cannabis-based medicine. *Cannabinoids as Therapeutics*, 231-263.

Hall, W. & Degenhardt, L. (2010). Adverse health effects of non-medical cannabis use--authors' reply. *The Lancet, 375*(9710), 197.

Hashibe, M., Morgenstern, H., Cui, Y., Tashkin, D. P., Zhang, Z. F., Cozen, W., et al. (2006). Marijuana use and the risk of lung and upper aerodigestive tract cancers: Results of a population-based case-control study. *Cancer Epidemiology Biomarkers & Prevention, 15*(10), 1829.

Iskedjian, M., Bereza, B., Gordon, A., Piwko, C., & Einarson, T. R. (2006). Meta-Analysis of cannabis based treatments for neuropathic and multiple sclerosis-related pain. *Current Medical Research and Opinion, 23*(1), 17-24.

Laberge, J. C. & Ward, N. J. (2004). Research note: Cannabis and driving—research needs and issues for transportation policy. *Journal of Drug Issues, 34*(4), 971-989.

Lakhan, S. E. & Rowland, M. (2009). Whole plant cannabis extracts in the treatment of spasticity in multiple sclerosis: A systematic review. *BMC Neurology, 9*(1), 59.

Leizer, C., Ribnicky, D., Poulev, A., Dushenkov, S., & Raskin, I. (2000). The composition of hemp seed oil and its potential as an important source of nutrition. *Journal of Nutraceuticals, Functional & Medical Foods, 2*(4), 35-53.

Liguori, A. (2007). Marijuana and driving: Trends, design issues, and future recommendations. In M. Earleywine, *Pot politics: Marijuana and the costs of prohibition.* New York: Oxford University Press, USA.

Liguori, A., Gatto, C. P., & Jarrett, D. B. (2002). Separate and combined effects of marijuana and alcohol on mood, equilibrium and simulated driving. *Psychopharmacology, 163*(3), 399-405.

Liguori, A., Gatto, C. P., Jarrett, D. B., Vaughn McCall, W., & Brown, T. W. (2003). Behavioral and subjective effects of marijuana following partial sleep deprivation. *Drug and Alcohol Dependence, 70*(3), 233-240.

Llewellyn, C. D., Linklater, K., Bell, J., Johnson, N. W., & Warnakulasuriya, S. (2004). An analysis of risk factors for oral cancer in young people: A case-control study. *Oral Oncology, 40*(3), 304-313.

Lowenstein, S. R. & Koziol-McLain, J. (2001). Drugs and traffic crash responsibility: A study of injured motorists in Colorado. *The Journal of Trauma, 50*(2), 313.

Lozano, I. (2001). The therapeutic use of cannabis sativa (L.) In Arabic medicine. *Journal of Cannabis Therapeutics, 1*(1), 63-70.

Luvone, T., Esposito, G., De Filippis, D., Scuderi, C., & Steardo, L. (2009). Cannabidiol: A promising drug for neurodegenerative disorders? *CNS Neuroscience & Therapeutics, 15*(1), 65-75.

Lydon, J., Teramura, A. H., & Coffman, C. B. (1987). UV-B radiation effects on photosynthesis, growth and cannabinoid production of two cannabis sativa chemotypes. *Photochemistry and Photobiology, 46*(2), 201-206.

Martin, B. R. & Wiley, J. L. (2004). Mechanism of action of cannabinoids: How it may lead to treatment of cachexia, emesis, and pain. *J Support Oncol, 2*(4), 305-314.

Mechoulam, R. & Ben-Shabat, S. (1999). From gan-zi-gun-nu to anandamide and 2-arachidonoylglycerol: The ongoing story of cannabis. *Natural Product Reports, 16*(2), 131-143.

MedicineNet. (2010). Definition of public health. Accessed 08/18/2010 from http://www.medterms.com/script/main/art.asp?articlekey=5120

Mortati, K. (2007). Case review-marijuana: An effective antiepileptic treatment in partial epilepsy? A case report and review of the literature. *Reviews in Neurological Diseases.*

Pate, D. W. (1994). Chemical ecology of cannabis. *Journal of the International Hemp Association, 1*(2), 31-37.

Pierre, J. M. (2010). Psychosis associated with medical marijuana: Risk vs. Benefits of medicinal cannabis use. *American Journal of Psychiatry, 167*(5), 598.

Ramaekers, J. G., Berghaus, G., van Laar, M., & Drummer, O. H. (2004). Dose related risk of motor vehicle crashes after cannabis use. *Drug and Alcohol Dependence, 73*(2), 109.

Rocha, F. C., Stefano, S. C., Haiek, R. D., Oliveria, L. M., & Da Silveira, D. X. (2008). Therapeutic use of cannabis sativa on chemotherapy-induced nausea and vomiting among cancer patients: Systematic review and meta-analysis. *European Journal of Cancer Care*, *17*(5), 431-443.

Rog, D. J., Nurmikko, T. J., Friede, T., & Young, C. A. (2005). Randomized, controlled trial of cannabis-based medicine in central pain in multiple sclerosis. *Neurology*, *65*(6), 812.

Ronald, S. (2010). Medical marijuana users in substance abuse treatment. *Harm Reduction Journal*, *7*(3).

Rosenblatt, K. A., Daling, J. R., Chen, C., Sherman, K. J., & Schwartz, S. M. (2004). Marijuana use and risk of oral squamous cell carcinoma. *Cancer Research*, *64*(11), 4049.

Schwartzberg, L. S. (2007). Chemotherapy-Induced nausea and vomiting: Clinician and patient perspectives. *J Support Oncol*, *5*(2 Suppl 1), 5-12.

Sidney, S., Quesenberry Jr, C. P., Friedman, G. D., & Tekawa, I. S. (1997). Marijuana use and cancer incidence (california, united states). *Cancer Causes & Control*, *8*(5), 722.

Stephens, R. S., Roffman, R. A., & Simpson, E. E. (1993). Adult marijuana users seeking treatment. *Journal of Consulting and Clinical Psychology*, *61*(6), 1100.

Sussman, S., Lisha, N., & Griffiths, M. (in press). Prevalence of the addictions: A problem of the majority or the minority. Evaluation & the Health Professions.

Sussman, S., Stacy, A. W., Dent, C. W., Simon, T. R., & Johnson, C. A. (1996). Marijuana use: Current issues and new research directions. *Journal of Drug Issues*, *26*, 695-734.

Tashkin, D. P. (1999). Effects of cannabis on the lung and the defenses against infection and cancer. *School Psychology International*, *20*, 23-37.

Taylor, D. R., Fergusson, D. M., Milne, B. J., Horwood, L. J., Moffitt, T. E., Sears, M. R., et al. (2002). A longitudinal study of the effects of tobacco and cannabis exposure on lung function in young adults. *Addiction (Abingdon, England)*, *97*(8), 1055.

Tomida, I., Azuara-Blanco, A., House, H., Flint, M., Pertwee, R. G., & Robson, P. J. (2006). Effect of sublingual application of cannabinoids on intraocular pressure: A pilot study. *Journal of Glaucoma*, *15*(5), 349.

Turcotte, D., Le Dorze, J. A., Esfahani, F., Frost, E., Gomori, A., & Namaka, M. (2010). Examining the roles of cannabinoids in pain and other therapeutic indications: A review. *Expert Opinion on Pharmacotherapy*, *11*(1), 17-31.

Van Dam, N. T. & Earleywine, M. (2010). Pulmonary function in cannabis users: Support for a clinical trial of the vaporizer. *International Journal of Drug Policy*, doi:10.1016/j.drugpo.2010.04.001

Wade, D. T., Robson, P., House, H., Makela, P., & Aram, J. (2003). A preliminary controlled study to determine whether whole-plant cannabis extracts can improve intractable neurogenic symptoms. *Clinical Rehabilitation*, *17*(1), 21.

Walsh, D., Nelson, K. A., & Mahmoud, F. (2003). Established and potential therapeutic applications of cannabinoids in oncology. *Supportive Care in Cancer*, *11*(3), 137-143.

Watson, S. J., Benson Jr, J. A., & Joy, J. E. (2000). Marijuana and medicine: Assessing the science base: A summary of the 1999 institute of medicine report. *Archives of General Psychiatry*, *57*(6), 547.

Wilcox, P. M., Fetting, J. H., Nettesheim, K. M., & Abeloff, M. D. (1982). Anticipatory vomiting in women receiving cyclophosphamide, methotrexate, and 5-FU (CMF) adjuvant chemotherapy for breast carcinoma. *Cancer Treatment Reports*, *66*(8), 1601.

In: Marijuana: Uses, Effects and the Law ISBN 978-1-61209-206-5
Editor: Andrea S. Rojas

Chapter 4

THE MEANINGS OF DRUG USE AND THEIR RELATIONS WITH MARIJUANA USE IN ADOLESCENCE

Michele Settanni*[*], *Fabrizia Giannotta, Silvia Ciairano, Donna Spruijt-Metz and Rob Spruijt
University of Turin, Department of Psychology, Turin, Italy

ABSTRACT

The goal of the present study was to explore the meanings of using drugs in adolescence and the relationship between these meanings and involvement in drugs. Participants were 208 adolescents (107 boys and 101 girls), aged 14-19 (mean age= 17.43, st.dev.= 1.55), attending two types of high school in Turin, Italy. Participants completed two questionnaires, one about involvement in drugs and other one about the reasons for having sex. Using confirmatory analyses, we found:

1. two dimensions of meanings for using drugs: Conformity and Self-affirmation, Coping;
2. the Coping meaning was related to both higher involvement in drug use and habitual use of drugs;

[*] Corresponding author's mailing address: Michele Settanni; Via Giuseppe Verdi 10, 10124; Torino, Italy.

Our findings suggest some degree of similarity between meanings of using drugs and of heavy drinking. Our findings also suggest that to reinforce the personal capabilities for facingstress and psychological discomfort might result in a more efficient strategy for preventing drug use with respect to other strategies; preventing substance use may also help for conforming to the behaviours of the other people and/or self-affirming one's own personality.

INTRODUCTION

Adolescence is a period of life characterized by many changes. The biological, cognitive, affective, and social modifications, which occur in this period, are related to developmental tasks that youths must accomplish. First, puberty provokes a profound physical and structural transformation. The body, as Coleman and Hendry (2000) argue, alters radically in size and shape. Consequently, youths might experience a period of clumsiness and self-consciousness as they attempt to adjust to this change. Moreover, sexual maturation entails a restructuring of the way in which adolescents view and approach the opposite sex, leading to the first romantic relationships (Brown, 1999). Secondly, the acquisition of hypothetical and deductive reasoning has implications in a wide range of behaviors and attitudes. Thought and action might be distinguished from one another independently and a time-perspective becomes possible, allowing individuals to think about the future. Furthermore, formal reasoning leads to increased maturity in relationships, related to the development of moral reasoning, as well as improvement in communication skills. Finally, all the mentioned changes cited above affect identity construction. Indeed, the individual's identity should adapt to the new role the adolescent will take on in society. One must become an adult; which implies being independent from one's family, able to create one's own family and to support oneself financially. Thus, all the tasks adolescents must face imply a deep commitment and re-adjustment of the self from youth to adulthood.

During this period, experimentation and identification processes are at work to accomplish the developmental tasks required (Grotevant and Cooper, 1986). These processes might lead to different outcomes though. For instance, one may experiment with new abilities by joining new sport teams, or by participating in structured or non-structured activities typical of this age (e.g. going to discos, church, the library, and the cinema). However, adolescents may also feel the need to experiment with risky behaviors, such as alcohol or drug use. Identification with one's parents can also be a positive way to become an adult. However, an overly precocious and complete identification with the adult world can lead adolescents to leave school too early in order to follow in the parents' path by going to work. Sometimes negative outcomes might be reversed. For instance, one might experiment with drugs (e.g. marijuana) on occasion, but this experimentation may be limited to the adolescent period without having irreversible consequences on the individual's adjustment. On the other hand, identification with deviant peers could lead to heavy drug use with consequent problems in other areas (e.g. school), which in turn limit the individual's possibilities for the future. Thus, normative processes can lead to different life trajectories: some are positive while others put the individual at risk.

Meanings and Motives for Risk Behaviours in Adolescence

Risk behaviours, then, might occur during this phase as a result of attempts to act normative with ones social group, or to cope with new developmental tasks. Following this line, Jessor and colleagues in their Problem Behavior Theory by Jessor (Jessor, Donovan and Costa, 1991) have suggested that risk behaviors might be interpreted as normative. That is, they are the result of relations between contextual factors and personality features at a given time. Moreover, either healthy or risk behaviors may serve the same function. Indeed, as individuals play an active role in their development, behavior is an action that seeks to accomplish a goal, which is meaningful for growth during adolescent transition. Consequently, different types of conduct might be carried out to accomplish similar aims; they are, as Silbereisen and Noack argue (1988), "functionally equivalent". For instance, one can show independence from adults by smoking cigarettes because it is something adults do not approve of; or by trying to use adult language to affirm one's position in front of adults. The choice between different behaviors depends on the interaction between personal resources, limits and the context, as postulated by Jessor in his model (Jessor, Donovan, Costa, 1991).

Consistently with Problem Behavior Theory, studies have shown that risk behaviours in adolescence might have positive consequences for youth, and then positive meanings. For instance, adolescents who drink alcohol seem to have more friends than the abstainers (Engels and ter Bogt, 2001). In addition, they are more likely to think that alcohol makes parties and social meetings more agreeable, and it eases contact with girls (Engels, Knibbe, de Vries, Drop and van Breukelen, 1999). A moderate use of marijuana in adolescence is related to a better psychological adjustment (Shedler and Block, 1990). Finally, researchers showed that some "experimental risk taking" permits the exploration of "adult-like" activities and is a way to develop social and psychological competence, autonomy and self-regulation (Silbereisen, Eyferth and Rudinger, 1986; Shedler and Block, 1990). Thus, problematic behaviours in adolescence might be experienced as a way to obtain something very positive in life.

Might the meaning or the reasons adolescents given to their conduct be related to the behaviour? Few studies have tried to focus on what adolescents think about risk behaviours and if this is related to their conduct. With respect to tobacco smoking, some studies showed that adolescents who felt smoking gave them energy and helped them to study smoke more than the others (Spruijt-Metz, Gallagher, Unger and Anderson-Johnson, 2004; 2005). Regarding sexual behaviors, Gebhardt, Kuyper and Greunswen, (2003) found that adolescents who had had sex to please their partners or to enhance mood were more likely to have casual partners. Also Cooper, Shapiro, and Powers (1998) found that having sex for coping motives was related to lower levels of sexual activity, but also to promiscuity (many partners, sex with strangers) but this was not necessarily connected to less protection. They also found out that when youth who ranked high on intimacy and enhancement motives were in casual relationships, they were less likely to protect themselves against both pregnancy and STDs. Our previous studies confirmed a relationship between meanings for sex and involvement in risky behaviors also in Italian youth (Giannotta, Ciairano, Spruijts and Spruits-Metz, 2009). We underlined cross sectionally that negative social meanings were related to a lack of protection in sexual intercourse, whereas trangressional meanings were related to lack of protection at the first sexual intercourse. Finally, regarding alcohol use, social motives have been found to be linked to moderate drinking, enhancement motives to heavy and binge drinking, coping motives to solitary and heavy drinking and to alcohol-related problems, and conformity motives, while less consistent, to drinking in social contexts, but also to heavy drinking (see Kuntsche, Knibbe, Gmel and Engels, 2005 for a review). Regarding Italian youth, we found out in a recent study that coping motives were positively related to the high consumption of all alcoholic beverages and to drunkenness; conformity motives were negatively related to high beer consumption and drunkenness, while experimentation-transgression motives were positively related to high alcopops consumption (Graziano, Bina, Giannotta and Ciairano, submitted). Thus, there is a widespread literature that attests the relation between sexual behavior, cigarettes and alcohol use and meanings that youth attribute to those behaviors.

Regarding the use of illicit drugs, literature presents some studies that investigate the relationships between drugs meanings and drug use. The majority of the research focused on ecstasy and methamphetamine, investigating their role in social parties, as raves parties or similar types of events. For instance, Hansen, Maycock, and Lower (2001) in a qualitative study with youth of ecstasy users pointed out that reasons to use ecstasy were to get: controlled freedom, a loss of inhibitions, affirmation of friendships and, a range of sensory feelings related to enjoyment and pleasure. Regarding marijuana use, again with a qualitative study, Lee and Kirkpatrick (2006) underlined that marijuana might be used to cope with the stresses of home and community life in a group of Southeast Asian Youth living in San Francisco. Finally, using Cooper's four motives (1998), Simons, Correia, Carey and Borsari (1998) showed that coping and enhancement motives were associated to increased levels of marijuana use, and that conformity motives were linked to more problems related to marijuana use, in adolescence. Thus, some studies have shown the importance of the motives and the meanings that youth gave to their behaviours to understand the style of consumption of illicit drugs.

Among different types of substances experimented in adolescence, marijuana is one of the first drugs that youth try on in Italy (Ciairano, van Schuur, Molinengo, Bonino and Miceli, 2008). Indeed, a recent ESPAD survey has just underlined that Italian youth marijuana users are higher than the average mean in Europe (Hibell *et al.*, 2009). Moreover, in the same report it came out that Italy has one of the highest proportions of high-risk users, compared to other European countries. Thus, cannabis use is a quite relevant issue for Italian adolescents and there is a need to understand what the determinants of this use are.

In spite of that, no studies exist that investigate the meaning of drug use in general, and of marijuana use in particular in Italian youth. This issue might be of particular relevance to intervene against the excessive use of this substance among Italian youth. Because meanings of behaviour are related to behaviors, changes in meanings of specific behaviors could provoke shifts in the behaviours. In our case, meanings of drug use may provide innovative avenues for effective intervention programs in youth people.

The first aim of our study was to understand the underlying dimensions of meanings to have drug in a youth population. As a theoretical starting point, we meshed the Theory of Meanings (Spruijt-Metz, 1999) and elements from the Problem Behavior Theory (Jessor, Donovan and Costa, 1991; Jessor, 1998). The Theory of Meanings of Behavior is based, in part, on Jessor's Problem Behavior Theory (Jessor, Donovan and Costa, 1991). Jessor and his colleagues found that risk behaviors, such as substance use and unprotected sex, can serve similar psychological function, or have similar personal meanings. One of these meanings is the transgression of societal and legal norms (Costa, Jessor, Donovan and Fortenberry, 1995). Therefore, according to the Jessor's theory in this study, we took into account the possible meaning of transgression for drug use. Finally, we also referred to both Cooper's (1994) categorization of drinking motives. Consequently, we expected to find four dimensions of meanings of drug use: (1) coping meanings, that is, drug as a way to manage negative emotions or problems; (2) conformity meanings, that is, drug as a way to be accepted in the peer group; (3) self-affirmation meanings, that is, drug as a way to show adulthood and independence; (4) transgressional meanings, that is drug use as a way to break the rules.

The second aim of our study was to examine the relationships between meanings of drug and life-time marijuana use. In keeping with previous works (Simons, Correia, Carey and Borsari, 1998), we expected conformity, self-affirmation and coping motives to be related to marijuana use. We also expected transgressional meanings to be related to higher consume of cannabis. Finally, we explored possible differences in endorsement of the various meanings of drug according to degree of implication in marijuana use (desultory or habitual). We expected habitual users to use more coping motives than the other users.

METHODS

Participants

Participants were 208 adolescents, aged 14-15 (13%, N = 27), 16-17 (38%, N = 79) and 18-19 (49%, N = 102), males (52%, N = 107) and females (48%, N = 101) attending three types of high schools in Turin (Italy): lyceum[1] (24%, N = 50), technical (35%, N = 73) and vocational school (41%, N = 85).

[1] In Italy, there are different paths for the secondary school with diverse specializations. Generally, they can be divided into lyceums (classical, scientific, linguistic, psycho-pedagogic, artistic schools) technical institutes (for accountants, surveyors, industrial

Procedure

Teacher and parental consent and adolescent assent were required in accordance with Italian law and the ethical code of the Italian Professional Psychologist Association. A random sample of public high schools from Turin city and surrounding representative of Nord Western Italy, stratified by type were invited to participate in the study and all schools contacted agreed to do so. Students within the schools, stratified by gender, were then randomly selected and all of them agreed to take part in the study. No incentives were offered. Questionnaires were administered by trained research staff during classroom time. The adolescents were assured of confidentiality and anonymity, and teachers left the classroom during completion of the surveys.

Measures

Meanings of Drug Use

We used the Questionnaire: ''My feelings about drugs'' (Ciairano, Bonino and Jackson, 1999). We conducted semi-structured interviews with 120 adolescents, 48% (N = 58) males and 52% (N = 62) females, 48% (N = 58) aged 14-17 years and 52% (N = 62) 18-19 years, to generate a list of possible meanings of drug use. The items in the questionnaire were based on these interviews as well as on theoretical considerations (Ciairano, 2004). The lead-in to the questions on meanings of drug use was: ''I am most likely to use drugs (as marijuana)'', followed by 15 possible meanings of drug use (see Table 1). The range of answers (closed answers) was from 1 = likely to be not correct to 5 = likely to be correct.

Involvement in Drug Use

We used the questions from the ''Io e la mia salute'' (Bonino, Cattelino and Ciairano, 2005), adaptated to the Italian context from the ''Me and my health'' Questionnaire (Jessor, Donovan and Costa, 1992) to assess the degree of involvement in drug use. These questions were: (1) Have you ever smoked a joint? (In case of affirmative response: yes, once, more than once); (2) Students who declared to having smoked were asked about their frequency of

---

technicians) and professional institutes (with different specializations ranging from artisan or secretarial and tourism to social care). All of these kinds of school allow access to university (see Bonino, Cattelino and Ciairano, 2006).

use in the last six months. We then recoded the answers to build up a typology of marijuana smokers, composed of the following categories: 1. Non users; 2. Stop (smoked marijuana but not in the last six months); 3. Desultory (smoked marijuana from 1 to 4-5 times in the last six months); 4. Habitual (smoked marijuana from once a month to every day)

Analyses

The statistical procedures we employed were different for the two aims of the study:

We used a combination of methods to obtain a statistical model for the underlying dimensions of meanings.

Table 1. Meanings of Drug use: items and factor loadings

Item		Factor	Factor loading from CFA
1.	To feel new sensations	-	-
2.	To prove that I am able to	1	.88
3.	To prove I am a man/woman	1	.98
4.	To escape the reality	2	.92
5.	To feel myself stronger	1-2	.50 - .44
6.	Because I do not feel self confident	2	.91
7.	Because I do not get on well with my parents	2	.93
8.	Because I am not well at school	2	.90
9.	To avoid making a bad impression with friends	-	-
10.	To tell friends	1	.96
11.	Because my friends have already tested it	1	.93
12.	To join a group of friends	-	-
13.	To share something dangerous with friends	-	-
14.	To share something exciting and new with friends	1	.77
15.	Because my parents wouldn't mind it	1	.91

(1) Dimensions of Meanings

To maximize the number of cases available for analyses we used PRELIS in LISREL 8.7 to impute missing values for case with a single missing value. Exploratory factor analysis (EFA) (PROMAX procedure in PRELIS) was used to evaluate possible two, three and four factor models. On the basis of EFA results, Confirmatory Factor Analysis (CFA) procedures were then used to formally specify the emerging model and to yield more informative fit measures.

We selected items for the CFA considering the factor loadings obtained from the exploratory procedures. The polychoric correlation matrix and the asymptotic covariance matrix generated by PRELIS was used as input to obtain parameter estimates for the chosen model, using the Weighted Least Squares method. This method was chosen because data were recorded on ordinal scales.

(2) Relations between Meanings and Behavior

After testing the model of meanings of drug use, we weighted the items by the factor scores' values and we summed up them in each dimension.

After computing the appropriate sum scores for the dimensions of meanings, the relation between dimensions of meaning of drug use and behavioral outcomes was examined using ANOVA, controlling for age and gender. Considering the sample size, we accepted as marginally significant a *p* values lower than .10.

RESULTS

Sample

Through imputation of missing values three cases were saved, yielding an effective sample size of 193.

In our sample, 56% (N = 75) has never smoked marijuana. Of the 44% who experienced marijuana use 9% did not smoke in the last 6 months, 14% were desultory users and 21% were habitual smokers.

Dimensions of Meanings

In the exploratory factor analysis three items were discarded as they produced Heywood cases (items #1, #9, #12 and #13, see table 1). The two factor model seemed more interpretable and more parsimonious than the three and the four factor model. Ten items fulfilled the requirements of sufficiently high loadings (> .45) and specificity (no loading on other factors above .30), while one item showed high loadings with both the extracted dimensions (item #5). On the basis of the content of the items, the two dimensions were tentatively labeled as 1. Conformity and Self affirmation; 2. Coping Meanings.

Subsequently, a structural model was specified with two interrelated dimensions and with only one item loading on both dimensions (item #5, to feel myself stronger) and without correlated errors. This model yielded good fit measures: Chi-square = 55.87, df=41, p = .06, RSMEA = .04, GFI = .99, NFI = 1.00. It appears that the two factor model of meanings of drug use describe the data well.

Involvement and Meanings of Drug Use

Our second aim was to test the relationship between meanings and involvement in drug use using univariate ANOVAs. Given that in previous analyses we found differences by gender and age, we controlled for the effect of the two variables in each analysis.

Involvement in Marijuana Use

The ANOVAs analyses was conducted using Involvement (never tried vs. having tried at least once) as independent variable and Coping and Conformity/Self affirmation factor scores as dependent variables in two separate analyses (see descriptive statistics in Table 2).

The Conformity/Self affirmation dimension showed no significant relation with involvement, while with Coping we found a significant effect of the involvement ($F\ (3,189)= 8.1$, $p<.05$, $\eta^2=.06$) with higher levels of the variable associated with students who tried to smoke at least once.

Table 2. Mean and standard deviation weighted sum score of behavioral measures on dimensions of meanings of drug use for Italian adolescents (ANOVA, controlling by age and gender)

		Conformity/Self affirmation M (SD)	Coping M (SD)
Involvement	Never	8.20 (3.78)	6.29 (3.53)[a]
	At least once	9.38 (3.36)	8.16 (3.94)[b]
Typology of marijuana users	Never	8.20 (3.78)	6.29 (3.53)[a]
	Stop	10.51 (5.05)	7.06 (3.06)[ab]
	Desultory	9.27 (3.02)	7.86 (3.29)[ab]
	Habitual	8.97 (2.65)	8.82 (4,59)[b]
	Whole sample	8.72 (3.64)	

Note: Different letters indicate significantly different mean values, with $p < .05$.

Tipology of Marijuana Users

Two ANOVA analyses were then conducted using Typology of Marijuana users as predictor and again factor scores as dependent variables (see Table 2). Even in this case we found no relationships between Conformity/Self affirmation and the independent variable. Instead, the second dimension showed to be significantly related to the different types of consumers ($F(3,189)=3.7$, $p<.01$, $\eta^2=.08$), with significant differences between Never users and Habitual users. In particular, Habitual users had the highest level of this variable.

Conclusions

On the bases of the Theory of Meanings (Spruijt-Metz, 1999), of the Problem Behavior Theory (Jessor, Donovan and Costa1991; Jessor, 1998), and of the categorization of drinking motives by Cooper's (1994), originally we expected to find four dimensions of meanings of drug use in a youth population: coping meanings, that is, drug as a way to manage negative emotions or problems; conformity meanings, that is, drug as a way to be accepted in the peer group; self-affirmation meanings, that is, drug as a way to show adulthood and independence; and finally, transgressional meanings, that is drug use as a way to break the rules. However, from this study only two dimensions emerged, that we labelled as Conformity and Self affirmation; and Coping Meanings. Thus, drug use seemed to not have a strong transgressional meaning for the adolescents who participated in the present study. This finding may be explained considering that the prevalence of drug use is about 30% in the interviewed participants. That is to say, that at least some experimentation with drug is almost normative in youth population. As a consequence, drug use does not seem to have a strong meaning of transgressing against adult norms, hence adolescents do not refer to this meaning in the interviews. Although this interpretation certainly needs further confirmation with wider and different groups of participants, it seems to support what Shedler and Block (1990) already underlined in their previous studies. Furthermore, differently from our expectations Conformity and Self affirmation, instead of being two separate dimensions, seems to represent two sides of the same coin. It is likely that the interrelationship between Conformity and Self affirmation refers to the strong connection between the processes of individuation and separation or differentiation in the development of identity. In fact, it is well known (Erickson, 1968) that adolescents have to accomplish both the processes of individuating with somebody (most likely the friends in the peer group) and of differentiating from somebody else (most likely the parents and other adults, but also peer groups different from one's own). These processes seem to be both present in adolescent drug use but differently from what we expected since they constitute a single dimension instead of two separate dimensions. It seems reasonable that this phenomenon is particularly evident in drug use rather than with different kinds of behaviour. This because adolescents may use substances similar or different from those used by their peers and/or they may use similarly or differently the same substance (that is, in a more or less frequent way, more or less quantity, individually or in a social context).

In our previous studies about meaning of sex (Giannotta, Ciairano, Spruijts and Spruits-Metz, 2009) and alcohol (Graziano, Bina, Giannotta and Ciairano, submitted) we found something different . For sex we found that negative social meanings were related to a lack of protection in sexual intercourse, trangressional meanings were related to lack of protection at the first sexual intercourse. For alcohol, we found that coping motives were positively related to the high consumption of all alcoholic beverages and to drunkenness; conformity motives were negatively related to high beer consumption and drunkenness, while experimentation-transgression motives were positively related to high alcopops consumption. Summarising, transgressional meaning seemed to be more related to a failure in accomplishing healthy behavior for protecting physical health and to some extent also in controlling one's own drinking (moderate drinking is normative in Italy, while heavy drinking is not; in fact we also found that conformity motives have a protective effect against heavy drinking), and coping meanings were related to both heavy drinking and drug use.

The second aim of our study was to examine the relationships between the personal meanings of drug and life-time marijuana use. In keeping with previous works (Simons, Correia, Carey and Borsari, 1998), we expected that Conformity and Self-affirmation and coping motives were related to marijuana use. Furthermore, we expected that the various meanings of drug reflect in different degrees of implication in marijuana use (desultory or habitual). More precisely, we expected that habitual users would use Coping motives more frequently than the other users. We did not find any relation between the Conformity/Self affirmation dimension and involvement, while we found a significant relationship between higher levels of the involvement and Coping meaning.

Furthermore, we found no relationship between different types of consumers and Conformity/Self affirmation. However, even in this case we found a significant difference with respect to Coping meaning: Habitual users quoted more often than Never users Coping meaning.

That is to say that the adolescent seemed more likely to use marijuana mainly as a coping strategy for facing discomfort instead of using it for conforming to the other people (presumably peers) and/or for affirming one's own individuality. Furthermore, the higher the frequency of use, the higher was also the use of marijuana for facing personal discomfort by the adolescents.

With respect to the lack of a relationship between Conformity/Self affirmation and marijuana use we can interpret it thinking that drugs, also the so-called soft drugs that are very common, are illegal in Italy. Probably this fact makes the adolescents more likely to find other more legal and/or socially accepted ways for identifying with the other people and/or for conforming to their behavior. For instance, adolescents may conform to the norms of the peer group not drinking alcohol (Graziano, Bina, Giannotta and Ciairano, submitted). Otherwise, they may conform to social norms by answering developmental tasks with adaptive behaviours such as studying for passing the exams at school and/or dating with a partner (Havirghurst, 1952). It is also noteworthy that using marijuana for Conformity/Self affirmation is neither related to use in general, nor to the type of use. Considering that in the case of drug use the meaning of Conformity/Self affirmation is likely to be interrelated with the peer group, it seems that the peer group and also the possibilities of affirming one's own identity in the eyes of peers is not enough for promoting marijuana use and/or becoming a habitual user. Although this finding certainly needs further confirmation in different and wider samples, the adolescents may need other more personal reasons for becoming involved in drug use. In the present study we found a strong relationship between drug use and the meaning of using drugs as a way of coping with psychological stress and discomfort. In a previous study we found that personal vulnerabilities (Ciairano, Settanni, Van Schuur and Miceli, 2006) were related to increasing levels of involvement at least at a longitudinal level. However, the present study was cross-sectional and we could not anticipate the direction of the relationship between coping and drug use. It might be that higher levels of discomfort and/or stress at time 1 predict drug use at time 2, but it might also be that higher levels of drug use at time 1 predict discomfort and/or stress at time 2. There are at least four non-alternative possible paths of this relationship.

On the one side and first becoming a drug user may also promote conflicts with one's own social context and thus also psychological discomfort and stress. Second, if the neuronal transmission is modified by the use of drugs and this is likely to affect also personal moods and feelings.

On the other side and third, people who feel high stress and discomfort may also be more likely to become a drug user and/or they may increase their level of use trying to face their own personal discomfort.

Furthermore we cannot forget that involvement in drugs is usually characterised in different steps (from approaching the use of substances to becoming a "hard" user; Ravenna, 1997), each one of them is likely to be characterised by a different meaning. That is, it would be interesting to follow each one of the different types of adolescent users at time 1 for checking which is the main meaning of drug use the same adolescents use most frequently at time 2; especially in the case of those who modify their style of use from desultory to habitual use. At the same extent some changes in the social context related to the changes in the style of use are also likely.

We also expected that transgressional meaning was related to higher consumption of cannabis. However, this relationship could not be explored because, as discussed earlier, we did not individuate any transgression meaning at least analysing the awareness of the adolescents about their involvement in substance use.

With respect to awareness, among all the other potential limitations, this study relied entirely on the meanings of drug use the adolescent were aware of and not on different and deeper meanings. Besides, the study had a cross-sectional design, which did not allow us to investigate the direction of the above mentioned relationships, as we anticipated earlier.

Finally, the findings are difficult to generalize to wider and different samples because they were drawn from a small group of participants of a particular European region, that is the North-West of Italy. Italy has some peculiarities with respect to the other western countries, such as longer transition to adulthood, greater centrality of the family in the success of adolescent developmental processes and the illegality of both the so-called light and hard drugs (Bonino, Cattelino and Ciairano, 2006).

However, despite these and other limitations we think that our findings represent another important piece of information in the field of studies that may inform the preventive intervention programs addressed to the adolescents. The following are the main strengths of the present study. First, it is one of the few studies that investigates the meanings adolescents attribute to drug use directly, taking into account their opinion, and not only indirectly by analysing the relationships between protective and risk factors and drug use behaviour. That is it is one of the few studies that takes into account the positive functions adolescent risk behaviours fulfil by helping them face their developmental tasks (Silbereisen and Noack, 1988).

Second, it is one of the few studies in this field within the Italian context, which is usually underrepresented, despite its potential interest because of the above mentioned Italian peculiarities. Finding similarities in the underlying processes of adolescent involvement in drug use between western countries with a different social and cultural contexts might be informative for establishing more efficient universal preventive strategies.

In the present study, we showed that to reinforce the personal characteristics of the adolescents and to help them in finding coping strategies more adaptive than using substances for facing stress and psychological discomfort might be more helpful than other kinds of interventions, such as teaching them not to conform to peer norms and not to affirm oneself by using drugs.

REFERENCES

Bonino S., Cattelino E., & Ciairano S. (2006). Italy. In Jeffrey J. Arnett (ed.), *International Encyclopedia of Adolescence*, 2 vols., New York-London: Routledge, 510-523.

Bonino S., Cattelino E., & Ciairano S. (2005). *Adolescents and risk. Behaviors, functions and protective factors.* New York: Springer Verlag.

Brown, B.B. (1999). "You are going out with whom?": Peer Group influences on Adolescent Romantic Relationship. In W. Furnam, B. Bradford Brown, & C. Feiring (Eds.). *The development of Romantic Relationship in Adolescence* (291-330). Cambridge: Cambridge University Press.

Ciairano, S. (2004). *Risk behaviour in adolescence: drug-use and sexual activity in Italy and the Netherlands.* Groningen (The Netherlands): Stichting Kinderstudies Publisher; avalaible; http://www.ub.rug.nl/eldoc/dis/ppsw/s.ciairano/thesis.pdf

Ciairano, S., Bonino, S., & Jackson, S. (1999). *Questionario: Io e i miei vissuti sull'uso di droga.* [*Me and my feelings about drugs*]. Department of Psychology, University of Groningen (The Netherlands).

Ciairano, S., Settanni, M., Van Schuur, W., & Miceli, R. (2006), Adolescent Substance Use, Resources and Vulnerabilities: A Cross-national and Longitudinal Study. *SUCHT, German Journal of Addiction Research and Practice, 52* (4), 253-260.

Ciairano, S., van Schuur, W. H., Molinengo, G., Bonino, S., & Miceli, R. (2008). Age of initiation with different substances and relationships with resources and vulnerabilities: a cross-national study. *European Journal of Developmental Psychology, 6,* 666-684.

Coleman, J.C., & Hendry, L.B. (2000). *The nature of adolescence (Third edition).* London, Routledge.

Cooper, M.L. (1994). Motivations for alcohol use among adolescents: development and validation of a four-factor model. *Psychological Assessment*, *6*, 117-128.

Cooper, M.L., Shapiro, C.M., & Powers, A.M. (1998). Motivations for sex and risky sexual behaviour among adolescents and young adults: A functional perspective. *Journal of personality and social psychology, 75,* 1528-1558.

Costa, F.M., Jessor, R., Donovan, J.E., & Fortenberry, J.D. (1995). Early initiation of sexual intercourse: the influence of psychosocial unconventionality. *Journal of Research on Adolescence, 5* (1), 93-121.

Engels, R. C., Knibbe, R. A., de Vries, H., Drop, M. J., & van Breukelen, G. J. (1999) Influences of parental and best friends' smoking and drinking on adolescent use: a longitudinal study. *Journal of Applied Social Psychology, 29,* 337–361.

Engels, R.C.M.E., & ter Bogt, T. (2001). Influences of risk behaviors on the quality of peer relations in adolescence. *Journal of Youth and Adolescence, 30 (6),* 675-695.

Erikson, E. H. (1968). *Identity: Youth and crisis.* Norton, New York.

Gebhardt, W.A., Kuyper, L., & Greunsven, G. (2003). Need for intimacy in relationships and motives for sex as determinants of adolescents condom use. *Journal of adolescent health, 33,* 154-164.

Giannotta, F., Ciairano, S., Spruijt, R., & Spruijt-Metz, D. (2009). Meanings of sexual intercourse for Italian adolescents. *Journal of Adolescence*, 32, 157-169.

Graziano, F., Bina, M., Giannotta, F., & Ciairano, S., Drinking motives and alcoholic beverage preferences among Italian adolescents, submitted to the *Journal of Adolescence.*

Grotevant, H.D., & Cooper, C.R. (1986). Individuation in family relationships: A perspective on individual differences in the development of identity and role-taking in adolescence. *Human development, 29,* 82-100.

Hansen, D., Maycock, B., & Lower, T. (2001). 'Weddings, parties, anything ... ', a qualitative analysis of ecstasy use in Perth, Western Australia. *International Journal of Drug Policy 12,* 181–199.

Havirghurst, R.J. (1952). Developmental tasks and education. Davis Mc Kay, New York.

Hibell, B., Guttormsson, U., Ahlström, S., Balakireva, O., Bjarnason T., Kokkevi A., & Kraus, L. (2009). *The ESPAD Report 2007. Alcohol and Other Drug Use Among Students in 35 European Countries.* Stockholm, Sweden: The Swedish Council for Information on Alcohol and Other Drugs.

Jessor, R. (ed.) (1998). *New perspectives on Adolescent Risk behavior.* New York: Cambridge University Press.

Jessor, R., Donovan, J.E., & Costa, F.M. (1991). *Beyond adolescence-problem behavior and young adult development.* New York: Cambridge University Press.

Jessor, R., Donovan, J.E., & Costa, F.M. (1992). *Health behavior Questionnaire. High School form.* Institute of Behavioral Science, University of Colorado Boulder, USA.

Kuntsche, E., Knibbe, R., Gmel, G., & Engels, R. (2006). "I drink spirits to get drunk and block out my problems...". Beverage preference, drinking motives and alcohol use in adolescence. *Alcohol & Alcoholism, 41*, 566-573.

Lee, J., & Kirkpatrick, S. (2006). Social meanings of marijuana use for Southeast Asian youth. *Journal of Ethnicity in Substance Abuse, 4*, 135–153.

Ravenna, M. (1997). *Psicologia delle tossicodipendenze.* Bologna: Il Mulino.

Shedler, J., & Block, J. (1990). Adolescent Drug Use and Psychological Health: A longitudinal Inquiry. *American Psychologist, 45,* 612-630.

Silbereisen, R.K., Eyferth, K., & Rudinger, G. (Eds.) (1986). *Development as action in context. Problem behavior and normal youth development.* Berlin: Springer-Verlag.

Silbereisen , R. K., & Noack, P. (1988). On the constructive role of problem behavior in adolescence. In A. Bolger, A. Caspi, G. Dolwney & M. Moorhose (eds.), *Person in context: Development process* (152-180). Cambridge: Cambridge University Press.

Simons, J., Correia, C.J., Carey, K.B., & Borsari, B.E. (1998). Validating a five-factor marijuana motives measure: relations with use, problems, and alcohol motives. *Journal of Counseling Psychology, 45,* 265–273.

Spruijt-Metz, D. (1999). *Adolescence, affect and health.* London, Psychology Press.

Spruijt-Metz, D., Gallaher, P., Unger, J., & Anderson-Johnson, C. (2004). Meanings of smoking and adolescent smoking across ethnicities. *Journal of Adolescent Health, 35,* 197–205.

Spruijt-Metz, D., Gallaher, P., Unger, J., & Anderson-Johnson, C. (2005). Unique contributions of meanings of smoking and outcome expectancies to understanding smoking initiation in middle school. *Annals of Behavioral Medicine, 30* (2), 104-111.

In: Marijuana: Uses, Effects and the Law
Editor: Andrea S. Rojas
ISBN 978-1-61209-206-5

Chapter 5

MARIJUANA AND ITS EFFECTS

Simone Fernandes and Taís de Campos Moreira
Universidade Federal de Ciências da Saúde de Porto Alegre, Porto Alegre, RS, Brazil

ABSTRACT

The consumption of Cannabis sativa held since 4000 BC being one of the first plants to be cultivated by man. Was recommend for prison-of-belly, malaria, rheumatism and also by adherents of some religions. Currently, marijuana is the most consumed illicit drug worldwide and the dependence is very common. In 2008, marijuana was used by 75.7 percent of current illicit drug users, in the USA. The effects and harm of marijuana use are well described and may involve physical effects such as tachycardia, dry mouth, dizziness, psychomotor retardation and psychological effects such as depersonalization, depression, anxiety, drowsiness and irritability. Chronic use complications can interfere with the operation of various systems such as pulmonary, reproductive and immune systems. The chronic user of marijuana may also submit amendments in relation to attention and the knee-jerk reactions. And these individuals may also report tolerance and withdrawal syndrome, as described in the literature. Marijuana is classified as a drug disturbing the central nervous system and its main psychoactive substance is the Δ-9-THC (tetrahydrocannabinol). After their consumption due to high lipid solubility, there is a change in the phospholipid membranes and the rapid action of THC on cannabinoid receptors. Few marijuana users seeking treatment for problem use of the substance and usually these individuals do not have the correct orientation of where to seek help. Pharmacological treatment for marijuana use and abstinence is not given and there are few studies on the subject. However it is known that psychosocial interventions are of great importance in the treatment to stop the use of marijuana.

INTRODUCTION

Historical and Origin

The origin of the world dissemination of the marijuana is associated to the use of the fiber of hemp in the making of fabrics and papers. The hemp is part of the Cannabis sativa plant (scientific name of the marijuana) that is native of the north region of the Afghanistan and it is between the first plant cultivated by the man for not alimentary ends. With the increase of the dissemination of the use of marijuana, were discovered his medicinal effects as the laxative effect of its seed, benefits against prison-of-belly, malaria, rheumatism and menstrual pains. Like this, many peoples passed consumed it also for medicinal ends, what caused to propagation of the benefits of consume it [1;2;3].

In the century XIX, the use of marijuana as psychotropic was restricted to small groups of people of the big cities and to the colonies of Asian immigrants and Africans situated in the West. In this epoch, the use of the substance was appropriate in the pharmacopeias official of several countries and medicines to base on marijuana could be bought in pharmacies. In the century XX, however, the scientists identified the side effects of the marijuana use and its use finished restrained or excluded in the pharmacopeias, being prohibited by law in several countries [4]. Nevertheless, in the years 60, the consumption of marijuana was increased very in the world.

The popular names of the marijuana pierced according to the preparations and countries in which are planted and traded. A weaker preparation, produced from the trial of drying of the sheets is called Bhang; Ganja is the given name to the strong preparation made with the flowers of the plants females; Charas is the more strong I prepare from the resin that covers the flowers females, also called of Hashish. To cannabis also is known as: marijuana, diamba, marijuana, pot, weed, grass, skunk, between others [2;5;4]. Today, in the

Holland, there is a politics of tolerance to the use of marijuana in the "coffee shops" of the big cities of the country [4;6;7], and, in some American states can be used with therapeutic ends [7]. In other regions around the world, the cultivation it, use it, transport it or sell it, it's considered illegal.

EPIDEMIOLOGY

Marijuana is the illicit drug more consumed around the world [8]. The number of individuals that experienced marijuana at least a time in 2008 in the world population, with age 15-64 years, was between 129 and 191 millions of people [9]. The dependence of marijuana is between the dependences of more common illicit drugs, 4.3 millions of people in the world used marijuana with consistent levels with abuse or dependence. [10]. It is to third drug more consumed for ends recreational in the U.S.A., staying behind barely of the consumption of alcohol and tobacco [11], being the illicit drug more utilized in the country [12]. It estimates itself that in 2020 they will be 5,7 millions of American north with age more than 50 illicit drugs users years, including marijuana [13]. The U.S.A. has presented a decrease in some age groups for the consumption of marijuana (Table1).

Table 1. Past month cannabis use by self- report, general US population

Age Group	2004	2005	2006	2007
12-17	7.6	6.8	6.7	6.7
18-25	16.1	16.1	16.3	16.4
26-29	10.8	9.9	10.1	9.8
30-34	6.4	7.6	7.0	6.3
35-39	5.2	4.9	5.8	5.4
40-44	5.7	4.7	5.3	4.5
45-49	5.1	4.8	4.8	4.9
50-54	3.8	3.7	4.1	3.8
55-59	1.7	2.5	1.3	2.1
60-64	0.2	0.9	1.5	0.6
≥ 65	0.1	0.3	0.2	0.2

Source: SAMHSA, Office of Applied Studies, National Survey on Drug use an Health

In the South America, although the annual predominance is minor that in the North America, around 3% of the population with age group between 15 and 64 years at least experienced marijuana in the year of 2008. The biggest marijuana consumption predominance in this region are in the Argentinean (7,2%), Chile (6,7%) and Uruguay (6%) [9]. In the Africa, in 2008, was observed an increase in the consumption of marijuana in comparison to the previous year. Approximately 26% to 58% of the patients attended in centers of handling specialized in the Africa related to consume cannabis [9]. In the Europe, around 29.5 millions of people (5,4%), with age between 15 and 64 years, consumed cannabis in 2007. The consumption of marijuana is widely concentrated between the youths (15-34 years). The Czech Republic (15.2% - 2008), Italy (14.6% - 2008) and Spain (10.1% - 2007) healthy the three countries with bigger predominance of consumers, being responsible by around a third of all of the consumers of cannabis in the Europe (5 millions barely in the Italy) [9].

Main Effects

The marijuana can produce effects as increase of the self-confidence, hilarity, sensation of relaxation and increase of the capacity of introspection. Beyond that, also complications occur that involve psychological and physical effects. The most common physical effects are tachycardia, dry mouth, dizziness, psychomotor delay and increase of the appetite; while the psychological effects appear like depersonalization, depression, anxiety, drowsiness, irritability and decrease in the attention. Some systems of the agency specially can be affected, as the pulmonary system, the reproductive system and the immunological system. Can occur still, important alterations regarding the and in the reaction of reflected [14;3;15;16]. For displayed newborns in the gestation to the use of marijuana made by the mother, there is answer neurobehavioral injured upon being born, beyond that, showed been irritated more and excited and less responsive to stimuli, what can influence substantially in the capacity of bond of the baby with its mother [17]. Like this, specially early the individual is displayed to the use of marijuana, bigger will be the damages caused to the health [18;19;20;21]. The consequences of these physical alterations project itself in the psychological, lawful, and social problems future of the infant. Many studies concern itself in show the as much as one the use of marijuana is associated to important psychosocial injury in the life of the individual [22]. Problems as loss of memory, little energy, procrastination, difficulty for sleep, by example, interfere substantially in activities of work and/or study. This can be cause to loss of job, family misunderstanding and, to even, to lawful problems, by be a matter of an illicit drug [22].

During some time to syndrome with the symptoms of the interruption of the use of marijuana was not described. This generated the idea of that there was not syndrome of abstinence, that the marijuana would cause minors injury and would not develop dependence [23; 24]. That fact did also with that did not develop specific handlings for the cessation of the use of marijuana [25]. However, symptoms of tolerance, the need of use bigger quantities of marijuana for obtain the same effects that before and syndrome of abstinence, have been shown in people that do daily use of big doses [26]. Individuals relate irritability, restlessness, diminution of the appetite, disturbances of the sleep, aggressive behavior and physical discomfort, as the main symptoms of abstinence caused by the discontinuity of the use of marijuana [25; 26;27].

Pharmacological Aspects of Marijuana Use

Marijuana Brazilian popular name of the plant Cannabis Sativa, Moraceae, features more than 400 components, of which approximately 60 of these components are cannabinoids [28]. The main cannabinoid is Δ^9-THC or THC, whose concentration in the plant Delta-9-tetrahydrocannabinol varies from 0.3% to 30%, which contributes to the variability of the THC levels in human tissues after the use of substance [29]. In humans, perceptual and motor speeds are faulty after use of a gram of marijuana containing 2% THC, which is considered a low dose for the consumption patterns [30].

Cannabis can be ingested as teas or be smoked, as a higher prevalence of use of this substance [31], or ingested with fatty foods, because of its lipophilic characteristics. Your use of intravenous form is not appropriate because the cannabis is not soluble in water [32]. When marijuana is smoked, THC is absorbed through the lungs, rapidly reaching the bloodstream. Its peak concentration is approximately 10 minutes after inhalation [33]. Presents 30% bioavailability, however, when ingested, gastrointestinal absorption of THC varies between 30-60 minutes, with this route, a reduction of bioavailability of the drug in 4-12% [34].

Due to the lipophilic characteristics of THC, the substance is rapidly distributed and stored in adipose tissue [33]. Therefore, there is slow release of THC from the body of adipocytes, resulting in half-life of about four days, according to the dose used [35].

After distribution to tissues, cannabis reaches the liver where it is metabolized by cytochrome P450 enzyme Δ and Δsystem, 11-hydroxy-9-tetrahydrocannabinol 8-hydroxy-9-tetrahydrocannabinol, both active metabolites [36, 37]. The second phase of metabolism has the end product is - 9-tetrahydrocannabinol-acyl-glucuronide (CTHC), the mainΔ11-nor-9-carboxy- metabolite found in urine and faeces [38].

The elimination of CTHC depends on the rate of biotransformation of precursor metabolites [39]. The half-life for elimination of this compound is approximately 6.2 days for non-frequent users of marijuana, and 5.2 days for frequent users [38]. The CTHC is a useful biological marker in the diagnosis of cannabis use, and are commonly identified by chromatography [40].

Marijuana is classified as a drug disturbing Central Nervous System (CNS) [41]. After consumption due to high doses THC, there is a change in the phospholipids of biological membranes, a phenomenon that enables quick action of THC on cannabinoid receptors in the CNS [42].

The cannabinoid receptors are inserted into the cell membrane, coupled to G protein and the enzyme adenylate cyclase, and are classified into two subtypes, according to their distribution [43, 44]. The type CB1 receptors predominate in the CNS and some peripheral nerve terminals, CB2 receptors are found mainly in immune cells such as lymphocytes and macrophages, associated with modulation of cytokine immune tissues [45, 46], but are also present in the CNS. Associated with these receptors are found endogenous ligands, endocannabinoids, classifieds, which include anandamide (araquid-onoiletanolamida) and 2-araquidonoil-glycerol [47, 42]. These substances are synthesized according to the physiological needs of the organism and subsequently removed from its site of action by the process of reuptake, is metabolized by intracellular enzymes [48]. Anandamide acts as a partial THC agonist of CB1 receptors, as well as the This leaves the endocannabinoid postsynaptic cells to activate the CB1 receptors in the presynaptic neuron [47]. In the CNS, the CB1 and CB2 receptors are found in several areas with specific functions, such as cerebellum and basal ganglia (responsible for motor coordination), hippocampus (learning and memory) and cortex (cognitive function) [43]. This distribution is related to the psychopharmacological effects of cannabis [49]. The receptors become active when they interact with ligands such as anandamide (endogenous agonist of cannabinoid receptors) or THC (exogenous agonist) [42]. This phenomenon triggers a series of reactions, such as G protein activation and inhibition of adenylate cyclase, which consequently reduces the production of cyclic AMP (cyclic adenosine monophosphate), important for cell homeostasis, opening of potassium channels and channel blockade calcium [41].

By acting on receptors, CB2, cannabinoid agonists promote hypotension and antinociception [50]. This phenomenon occurs due to indirect interaction with the opioid system, especially with kappa opioid receptors, a phenomenon that explains the sensation of analgesic effects after use of marijuana [51].

A peculiarity of cannabinoid receptors relates to their location in the presynaptic membrane, indirectly influencing several neurotransmitter systems such as gamma-aminobutyric acid (GABA), glutamate, norepinephrine, serotonin and dopamine [52]. On glutamatergic neurotransmission and noradrenergic, cannabinoid receptors act by inhibiting calcium channels and activate potassium channels, promoting a block in the release of these neurotransmitters. Another significant mechanism of THC is via its action on endogenous opioids, which under the effect of exogenous agonist; indirectly stimulate the dopaminergic system, promoting positive reinforcement after using the substance [53].

Treatment for Cessation Marijuana Use

Few marijuana users seeking treatment for their problematic use. Usually do not have guidance on where to seek help or what kind of treatment is most appropriate. This is justified by the fact that for a long time believed that marijuana does not cause withdrawal symptoms or dependency [23, 24]. Thus, having no specific treatment for marijuana users, the number of individuals receiving treatment is much lower than other drugs such as cocaine, for example [54, 55]. Pharmacological treatment for marijuana use is still uncertain and there are few studies on the subject [54]. The increase in dopaminergic transmission in the nucleus accumbens (NAc) by acute administration of cannabinoid agonists can be blocked with the use of cannabinoid CB1 antagonist. Thus, cannabinoid CB1 antagonists may be an alternative to treatment for marijuana use. The best known is Rimonabant (SR 141716A), a medication developed for obesity and that has been used in research for treatment of tobacco use and marijuana [54, 55, 47].

Human studies have shown that abstinence can be observed in the abrupt cessation of heavy use of cannabis or daily [56, 57], and there are a large number of marijuana users who have relapsed on stopping [55]. Therefore, there are some alternatives to the pharmacological withdrawal phase that have been studied the longest. It is known, in studies with rats, clonidine (α2 receptor agonist), decreases withdrawal symptoms by decreasing the output (output) noradrenergic, since there is strong evidence on the role of noradrenergic hyperactivity in the mediation of the withdrawal syndrome . However, due to adverse effects such as hypotension and sedation, another agonist of α2, the lofexidine may be more suitable for human trials [54, 58]. The readministration of delta-9-THC orally when withdrawal symptoms were precipitated by CB1 antagonist, has also proved a good strategy for the treatment of marijuana withdrawal syndrome [58], the use of prostaglandin E2, an end product of arachidonic acid cascade effect, attenuated withdrawal symptoms [59], and lithium, known mood stabilizer, was effective in preventing symptoms of withdrawal from marijuana as anxiety, depression and irritability in rats, acting on systemic oxytocin [60]. However, oxytocine can cause discomfort peripheral because it produces effects similar to those caused by benzodiazepines. Thus, an alternative would be to evaluate the effects of benzodiazepines such as clonazepam and oxazepam, (with less potential for addiction) in the marijuana withdrawal syndrome in humans [54]. The treatment of addiction in general, is increasingly focused on the idea of secondary prevention. In this context, brief interventions have increasingly been developed [61]. A brief motivational intervention (IBM) is an approach adapted from motivational interviewing for use in brief contacts in primary health care health [62] and is based on the stages of change model [63]. It is a technique of short duration that can be used by professionals not specializing. The strategies used to assess the stage of readiness to change, advise the individual as identified stage of change, working to provide ambivalence and self-help materials [64, 65, 66, 67]. The intervention is based on the individual and personalized, offers strategies that are related to minimizing the damage caused by drugs [61]. Besides being used in primary health care health, IBM has also been offered through phone calls [68, 69] together with supporting materials [70]. Using this approach with marijuana users have shown significant efficacy [71]. An important factor in IBM's assessment of motivation, it is useful to perform the appropriate action for the stages of change in which the individual can be. For example, individuals in the precontemplation stage should be helped to recognize and develop awareness of their problem rather than being directly guided to abstinence. Moreover, in the contemplation stage are open to interventions that increase awareness, but the guidelines are tough policies for action. In the action stage, clients need practical help with procedures for behavioral change [72].

There is a large number of patients that need services of primary health care, one of the reasons that made the phone were to become a good alternative to meet this demand effectively and with quality in the care [73]. Telemedicine is a new form of assistance and provision of health service to people because it enables the making targeted interventions to the problems of who accesses a specialized telephone service [74].

Applying the issue of drugs, many users do not know the treatment options or do not know how to get it. Due to the stigma around drug users, one anonymous and telephone service, such as helplines may be useful. The helplines are offered motivational materials, brief counseling and other services. Some studies show that this type of care is useful for tobacco cessation. There are helplines, too, for cocaine, marijuana, heroin and alcohol [75]. However, until now the efficiency / effectiveness of telephone services in Brazil were not assessed for abuse of marijuana, which makes the present study, is unprecedented. Although marijuana is the illicit drug most widely used and its use is associated with significant psychosocial problems, there are not many studies on the treatment of cannabis use [76, 8], and between them, the interventions did not vary much. Basically studying the use of cognitive-behavioral therapy and brief intervention using motivational interviewing (IBM), compared to minimal intervention (support materials). In all studies, the cognitive-behavioral therapy and IBM show better results compared to the control group [77, 8, 78].

Usually IBM also has a monitoring period to the user. This is because drug use in general and consequently also in the use of marijuana, having a monitoring period so that we can monitor the use can help stop the withdrawal final. Thus, most studies on the treatment of marijuana use have proposed the follow-up (follow-up) of patients in order to support the process of cessation of abuse. The levels of success have said that the closer the intervention, the better the success in being without using drugs and that success in segments of six months can reach 50% [78]. The IBM technical and cognitive behavioral therapies have proven effective in stopping the use of marijuana [8, 78, 79]. When comparing 14 sessions of cognitive-behavioral therapy, or a longer intervention, the two sessions of IBM, the success rate was very similar. This shows the effectiveness of IBM in relation to cognitive-behavioral therapy for cannabis use [78], since it has shorter duration. It also produces better results for the cessation of marijuana use than minimal interventions and their results are also favorable to reducing the occupational and psychosocial problems related to the drug [78].

CONCLUSION

Being a drug that became popular between controversies about beneficial use or harmful use, marijuana awaken it seems less interest to researchers and for this reason, a popular imagination was created about that causes less damage to those who use it. However, its consumption has been growing in recent years [80] and its users often do not know how, where and what treatment seeking [23]. This might be associated with the absence of specific treatments for marijuana dependence, because programs are often aimed at users of alcohol, cocaine or other drugs [77]. When marijuana users seeking treatment, they report substantial losses psychosocial adverse consequences related to the use, failure in attempts to stop the consumption and yet, self-perception of being unable to cease use [8, 78].

Although knowledge about the effects and harm of marijuana use has increased in recent years, there is still much to study. Once each year an increasing number of users and addicts of this drug, which still consider marijuana a drug that does not cause health problems. Efficient and effective treatments to be tested and offered to the entire population. Furthermore, the increase is necessary for campaigns to educate about the harm that marijuana can cause.

REFERENCES

[1] Russo EB. History of cannabis and its preparation in saga, science and sobriquet. *Chemistry & Biodiversity* 2007; 4: 1614-1698.

[2] Zuardi AW. History of cannabis as a medicine: a review. *Revista Brasileira de Psiquiatria* 2006; 28: 153-157.

[3] Crippa JA; Lacerda AL; Amaro E; Bussatto Filho G; Zuardi AW; Bressan RA. Brain effects of cannabis- neuroimaging findings. *Revista Brasileira Psiquiatria* 2005; 27: 70-78.

[4] CEBRID - *Centro Brasileiro de Informações sobre Drogas. Folhetos informativos sobre drogas psicotrópicas.* Departamento de Psicobiologia da UNIFESP [serial on line] 2007. Avaliable from: URL: http://www.unifesp.br/dpsicobio/cebrid/folhetos/maconha_.htm.

[5] NIDA – National Institute on Drug Abuse. *Marijuana.* National Institute on Drug Abuse [serial on line] 2007. Avaliable from: URL: http://www.nida.nih.gov/DrugPages/Marijuana.html.

[6] CENPRE – *Centro Regional de Estudos, Prevenção e Recuperação de Dependentes Químicos [serial on line] 2007.* Avaliable from: URL: http://www.cenpre.furg.br/maconha/hist_maco.htm.

[7] Carneiro H. *Pequena enciclopédia da história das drogas e bebidas.* Rio de Janeiro (RJ): Elsevier; 2005.

[8] Budney AJ; Higgins ST; Radonovich KJ; Novy PL. Adding voucher-based incentives to coping skills and motivational enhancement improves outcomes during treatment for marijuana dependence. *Journal of Consulting and Clinical Psychology* 2000; 68: 1051-1061.

[9] UNODC - United Nations Office on Drugs and Crime. *Word Drug Report 2010;* New York (N.Y).

[10] SAMHSA - Substance Abuse and Mental Health Services Administration [serial on line] 2006. Results from the 2005 National Survey on Drug Use and Health: National findings. *U.S. Department of Health and Human Services.* [cited 2007 Jun 5];1(1):[about 24 screens]. Available from: URL: http://www.samhsa.gov.

[11] Murray RM; Morrison PD; Henquet C; DiForti M. Cannabis, the mind and society: The hash realities. *Nat Rev Neurosci* 2007; 8: 885–95.

[12] Han B; Gfroerer JC; Colliver JD. Associations Between Duration of Illicit Drug Use and Health Conditions: Results from the 2005–2007 National Surveys on Drug Use and Health. *Annals of Epidemioly* 2010; 20: 4: 289-97.

[13] Han B; Gfroerer JC; Colliver J D; Penne MA. *Substance use disorder among older adults in the United States in 2020. Addiction 2009; 104: 88-96.*

[14] Ribeiro M; Marques ACPR; Laranjeira R; Alves HNP; Araújo MR; Baltieri DA et al. Abuso e dependência da maconha: diretrizes em foco [serial on line]. *Associação Médica Brasileira e Conselho Federal de Medicina 2005.* Avaliable from: URL: www.projetodiretrizes.org.br

[15] Babor TF. Brief treatments for cannabis dependence: findings from a randomized multisite trial. *Journal of Consulting and Clinical Psychology* 2004; 72: 455-466.

[16] Kalant H. Adverse effects of cannabis on health: an update of the literature since 1996. *Progress in Neuro-Psychopharmacology and Biological Psychiatry* 2004; 28: 849-863.

[17] Barros MCM; Guinsburg R; Peres, CA; Mitsuhiro S; Chalem E; Laranjeira R. Exposure to marijuana during pregnancy alters neurobehavior in the early neonatal period. *The Journal of Pediatrics* 2006; 149: 781-787.

[18] Arsenault L; Cannon M; Poulton R; Murrey R; Caspi A; Moffit TE. Cannabis use in adolescence and risk for adult psychosis: longitudinal prospective study. *British Medical Journal* 2002; 325: 1212-1213.

[19] Fergusson D; Swain-Campbell NR; Horwood LJ. Deviant peer affiliations, crime and substance use: a fixed effects regression analysis. *Journal of Abnormal Child Psychology* 2002; 30: 419–430.

[20] Stefanis NC; Delespaul P; Henquet C; Bakoula C; Stefanis CN; Van OJ. Early adolescent cannabis exposure and positive and negative dimensions of psychosis. *Addiction* 2004; 99: 1333-1341.

[21] Jungerman FS; Laranjeira R. Maconha: qual a amplitude de seus prejuízos? *Revista Brasileira de Psiquiatria* 2005; 27: 5-6.

[22] Stephens RS; Babor TF; Kadden R; Miller M. Marijuana treatment project (MTP). The marijuana treatment project: rationale, design, and participant characteristics. *Addiction* 2002; 97: 109-124.

[23] Macleod J; Oakes R; Copello A; Crome, I; Egger M; Hickman M et al. Psychological and social squeals of cannabis and other illicit drug use by young people: a systematic review of longitudinal, general population studies. *Lancet* 2005; 15: 363, 1579-88.

[24] Kleber HD. Future advances in addiction treatment. *Clinical Neuroscience Research* 2005; 5: 201-205.

[25] Budney AJ; Novy PL; Hughes JR. Marijuana withdrawal among adults seeking treatment for marijuana dependence. *Addiction* 1999; 94: 1311-1321.

[26] Haney M; Ward AS; Comer SD; Foltin RW; Fischman MW. Abstinence symptoms following smoked marijuana in humans. *Psychopharmacology* 1999; 141: 395-404.

[27] Vandrey RG; Budney AJ; Moore BA; Hughes JR. A cross-study comparison of cannabis and tobacco withdrawal. *American Journal on Addiction* 2005; 14: 54-63.

[28] Ribeiro M ; Marques ACPR; LARANJEIRA, R. et al. Abuso e Dependência da Maconha. *Revista da Associação Médica Brasileira* 2005; 51: 241-55.

[29] Honório KM; Arroio A; Silva ABF. Aspectos terapêuticos de compostos da planta *Cannabis sativa. Química Nova 2006*; 29: 2: 318-25.

[30] Kurzthaler I; Hummer M; Miller C; Sperner-Unterweger B; Günter V; Wechdorn H et al. Effect of cannabis use on cognitive functions and driving ability. *The Journal of Clinical Psychiatry* 1999; 60: 395-399.

[31] Gustafson RA; Levine B; Stout PR; Klette KL; George MP; Moolchan ET et al. Urinary Cannabinoid Detection Times after Controlled Oral Administration of Delta-9-Tetrahydrocannabinol to Humans. *Clinical Chemistry* 2003; 49: 7: 1114–1124.

[32] ASHTON, C.H. Pharmacology and effects of cannabis: a brief review. *British journal of psychiatry* 2001; 178:101-106.

[33] Johansson E; Noren K; Sjovall J; Halldin MM. Terminal elimination plasma half-life of delta 1-tetrahydrocannabinol (delta 1-THC) in heavy users of marijuana. *European Journal of Clinical Pharmacology* 1989a; 37: 273–277.

[34] Grotenhermen F. Pharmacokinetics and pharmacodynamics of cannabinoids. *Clinical Pharmacokinetics* 2003; 42: 327-360.

[35] Johansson E; Noren K; Sjovall J; Halldin MM.. Determination of delta 1 tetrahydrocannabinol in human fat biopsies from marihuana users by gas chromatography–mass spectrometry. *Biomedical Chromatography* 1989b; 3: 35–38.

[36] Watanabe K; Narimatsu S; Yamamoto I; Yoshimura H. Oxygenation mechanism in conversion of aldehyde to carboxylic acid catalyzed by a cytochrome P-450 isozyme. *Journal of Biological Chemistry* 1991; 266: 2709–2711.

[37] Deustch DG; Chin S. A. Enzymatic synthesis and degradation of anandamide, a cannabinoid receptor agonist. *Biochemical Pharmacology* 1993; 46: 791–796.

[38] Glaz-Sandberg A. Pharmacokinetics of 11-nor-9-Carboxy-D9-Tetrahydrocannabinol (CTHC) After Intravenous Administration of CTHC in Healthy Human Subjects. *Clinical Pharmacology Therapeutics* 2007; 82: 63-69.

[39] Hunt CA; Jones RT. Tolerance and disposition of tetrahydrocannabinol in man. *The Journal of Pharmacology and Experimental Therapeutics* 1980; 215: 35–44.

[40] Costantino A; Schwartz RH; Kaplan P. Hemp oil ingestionn causes positive urine tests for _9-tetrahydrocanabinol carboxylic acid. *Journal of Analytical Toxicology* 1997; 21: 482–5.

[41] Joy JE; Watson SJ; Benson J. A. Marijuana and medicine: assessing the science base: a summary of the 1999 Institute of Medicine Report. *Archives of General Psychiatry* 2000; 57: 547-552.

[42] Pertwee RG. Pharmacological Actions of Cannabinoids. In: *Handbook of experimental pharmacology - Cannabinoids.* Springer Berlin Heidelberg 2005. P. 1-151.

[43] Herkenham M; Lynn AB; Johnson M.; Melvin LS; Costa BR; Rice KC. Characterization and localization of cannabinoid receptors in rat brain: A quantative in vitro autographic study. *The Journal of Neuroscience* 1991; 11: 563–583.

[44] Munro S; Thomas KL; Abu-sahaar M. Molecular characterization of a peripheral receptor for cannabinoids. *Nature* 1993; 365: 61–64.

[45] Ihenetu K; Molleman A; Parsons M; Whelan C. Pharmacological characterization of cannabinoid receptors inhibiting interleukin 2 release from human peripheral blood mononuclear cells. *European Journal Pharmacology* 2003; 464: 207-15.

[46] Pertwee RG. Pharmacology of cannabinoid receptor ligands. *Current Medical Chemistry* 1999; 6: 635–664.

[47] Piomelli D. The endogenous cannabinoid system and the treatment of marijuana dependence. *Neuropharmacology* 2004; 47: 359-367.

[48] De Petrocellis L; Cascio MG; Di Marzo V. The endocannabinoid system: a general view and latest additions. *British Journal of* Pharmacology 2004; 141: 765–774.

[49] Pertwee RG. The evidence for the existence of cannabinoid receptors. *General Pharmacology* 1993; 24: 811–824.

[50] Calignano A; La Rana G; Piomelli D. Antinociceptive activity of the endogenous fatty acid amide, palmitoylethanolamide. *European Journal of Pharmacology* 2001; 419: 191–198.

[51] Welch SP; Huffman JW; Lowe J. Differential Blockade of the Antinociceptive Effects of Centrally Administered Cannabinoids by SR141716A1. *The Journal of Pharmacological and Experimental Therapeutics* 1998; 286: 1301–1308.

[52] Schlicker E; Kathman M. Modulation of transmitter release via presynaptic cannabinoid receptors. *Trends in Pharmacological Science 2001; 22: 565-72.*

[53] Chen J; Paredes W; Lowinson JH; Gaedner EL. Delta-9-tetrahydrocanabinol enhances presynaptic dopamine efflux in medial frontal cortex. *European Journal of Pharmacology* 1990; 190: 259-62.

[54] Hart CL. Increasing treatment options for cannabis dependence: a review of potencial pharmacotherapies. *Drug and alcohol dependence* 2005; 80: 147-159.

[55] Szabo B; Siemens S; Wallmichrath I. Inhibition of GABAergic neurotransmission in the ventral tegmental area by cannabinoids. *European Journal of Neuroscience* 2002; 15: 2057-2061.

[56] Budney AJ; Hughes JR; Moore BA; Novy PL. Marijuana abstinence effects in marijuana smokers maintained in their home environment. *Archives of General Psychiatry* 2001; 58: 917-924.

[57] Hart CL; Haney M; Ward AS; Fischman MW; Foltin RW. Effects of oral THC maintenance on smoked marijuana self-administration. *Drug and Alcohol Dependence 2002*; 67: 301-309.

[58] Lichtman AH; Fisher J; Martin BR. Precipitated cannabinoid withdrawal is reversed by delta(9)-tetrahydrocannabinol or clonidine. *Pharmacology, Biochemistry and behavior* 2001; 69: 181-188.

[59] Anggadiredja K; Yamaguchi T; Tanaka H; Shoyama Y; Watanabe S; Yamamoto T. Prostaglandin E2 attenuates SR141716A-precipitated withdrawal in tetrahydrocannabinol-dependent mice. *Brain Research* 2003; 14: 47-53.

[60] Cui SS; Bowen RC; Gu GB; Hannesson DK; Yu PH; Zhang X. Prevention of cannabis withdrawal syndrome by lithium: involvement of oxytocinergic neuronal activation. *The Journal of Neuroscience* 2001; 21: 9667-9876.

[61] Mccambridge J; Strang. The efficacy of single-session motivacional interviewing in reducing drug consumption and perceptions of drug-related risk and harm among young people: results from a multi-site cluster randomized trial. *Addiction* 2004; 99: 39-52.

[62] Rollnick S; Heather N; Bell A. Negotiating Behaviour Change in Medical Settings: the development of brief motivational interviewing. *Journal of Mental Health* 1992; 1: 25-37.

[63] Prochaska JO; Diclemente CC; Norcross JC. In search of how people change: applications to addictive behaviors. *The American Psychologist* 1992; 47: 1102-1114.

[64] Butler CC; Rollnick S; Cohen D; Bachman M; Russel I; Stott N. Motivational consulting versus brief advice for smoker in general practice: a randomized trial. *British Journal of General Practice* 1999; 49: 611-616.

[65] Miller WR; Rollnick S. *Motivational interviewing: preparing people for change*. 2sd ed. Porto alegre: Artmed, 2002.

[66] TevyamTO; Monti PM. Motivacional Enhancement and Other Brief Interventions for Adolescent Substance Abuse: Foundations, Aplications and Evaluations. A*ddiction* 2004; 99: 63-75.

[67] Tracy O, Peter M. Motivacional Enhancement and Other Brief Interventions for Adolescent Substance Abuse: Foundations, *Aplications and Evaluations. Addiction* 2004; 99: 63-75.

[68] Ramelson HZ; Friedman RH; Ockene JK. An automated telephone-based smoking cessation education and counseling system. *Patient Education Counseling* 1999; 36: 131-144.

[69] Lancaster T; Stead LF. Self-help Interventions for Smoking Cessation. Cochrane Database of Systematic Reviews [Online], v.3, 2005. Avaliable from: URL: http://mrw.interscience. wiley.com/ cochrane/ clsysrev/articles/CD001118/frame.html

[70] Britt E; Hudson SM; Blampied NM. Motivational interviewing in health settings: a review. *Patient Education and Counseling* 2004; 53: 147-155.

[71] Fernandes S; Ferigolo M; Benchaya MC; Moreira TC; Pierozan P.S; Mazoni CG et al. Brief motivational intervention and telemedicine: a new perpective of treatment to marijuana users. *Addictive Behaviors* 2010; 35: 750-755.

[72] Diclemente CC; Prochaska JO; Fairhurst SK; Velicer WF; Velasquez MM; Rossi JS. The process of smoking cessation: an analysis of precontemplation, contemplation, and preparation stages of change. *Journal of Consulting and Clinical Psychology*1991; 59: 295-304.

[73] Zhu SH; Stretch V; Balabanis F; Rosbrook B; Sadler G. Telephone counseling for smoking cessation: Effects of single-session and motivational interventions. *Journal of Consulting Clinical Psychology* 1996; 65: 202-211.

[74] Friedman RH; Stollerman JE; Mahoney DM; Rozenblyum L. The virtual visit: using telecommunications technology to take care of patients. *Journal of the American Medical Informatics Association* 1997; 6: 413-425.

[75] Hughes J; Riggs R; Carpenter M. How Helpful are Drug Abuse Helplines? *Drug and Alcohol Dependence* 2001; 62:191-194.

[76] Denis C; Lavie E; Fatséas M; Auriacombe M. Psychotherapeutic interventions for cannabis abuse and/or dependence in outpatient settings. Cochrane Database of Systematic Review [online] 2006; 3: CD005336: Avaliable from: URL: http://mrw.interscience. wiley.com/ cochrane/clsysrev/articles/CD005336/frame.html

[77] MTP (Marijuana Treatment Project Research Group). Brief treatments for cannabis dependence: findings from a randomized multisite trial. *Journal of Consulting and Clinical Psychology* 2004; 72: 455-466.

[78] Stephens RS; Roffman RA; Curtin L. Comparison of extended versus brief treatments for marijuana use. *Journal of Consulting and Clinical Psychology* 2000; 68: 898-908.

[79] Copeland J; Swift W; Rees V. Clinical profile of participants in a brief intervention program for cannabis use disorder. *Journal of Substance Abuse Treatment* 2001; 20: 45-52.

[80] Galduroz JCF; Noto AR.; Fonseca AM; Carlini EA. V *Levantamento sobre consumo de drogas psicotrópicas entre estudantes do ensino fundamental e médio da rede pública de ensino nas 27 capitais brasileiras.* São Paulo (SP): Centro Brasileiro de Informações sobre drogas psicotrópicas - CEBRID; 2004.

In: Marijuana: Uses, Effects and the Law
Editor: Andrea S. Rojas
ISBN 978-1-61209-206-5

Chapter 6

PSYCHOLOGICAL AND SOCIAL PREDICTORS OF MARIJUANA USE AMONG ITALIAN ADOLESCENTS: A ONE-YEAR FOLLOW-UP INVESTIGATION

Enrique Ortega and Silvia Ciairano***
University of Turin, Department of Psychology, Turin, Italy

ABSTRACT

In Italy the use of certain substances such as alcohol are encouraged and even guided by the family during adolescence, while others such as marijuana are strictly prohibited. Italian adolescents are among the highest in Europe for high-risk marijuana consumption. We investigated the one year longitudinal influence of our samples' personal (depression, stress, aggression, sensation seeking, and risk taking), family (strict family rule and parent approval of marijuana use), peer (peer approval of marijuana use and peer marijuana use) and school (academic marks) domains on three marijuana use indicators: lifetime use, past six month use frequency, and intoxication.

---

* Corresponding author's mailing address: Enrique Ortega Via Guiseppe Verdi 10, 10124 Torino, Italy

Research was conducted in the Italian province of Turin which is situated in Northern Italy. A sample of public high schools stratified by school type was invited to participate. The sample consisted of 324 youths (56% male) ranging in age from 15-20 (*M* = 17.29 yrs, *SD* = 1.61) living in northwest Italy and was reasonably balanced for gender (52% boys, 48% girls), and age (mean age = 17.4).

One year follow up analyses revealed that higher indications of depression at baseline were associated with lower indications of marijuana use at one year follow up (β = -0.24, p = 0.03), and with greater indications of marijuana use in the past six months (β = 2.66, p = 0.004). Similarly higher indications of sensation seeking at baseline were negatively associated with lifetime marijuana use at 1 year follow up (β = -0.010, p = 0.008). Higher indications of stress at baseline were associated with higher indications of lifetime marijuana use at follow up (β = 0.14, p = 0.03). Lastly, a greater perception of strict family rules at baseline was associated with lower indications of lifetime marijuana use (β = -0.32, p = 0.005) and with lower indications of past six month marijuana use frequency at 1 year follow up (β = -1.54, p = 0.02). Moderation analyses revealed a significant gender interaction between the association of sensation seeking and lifetime marijuana use (β = 0.23, p = 0.004).

This study represents a first attempt to uncover the marijuana use determinants of Italian adolescents. While not every important explaining factor has been studied here we have attempted to look at the effects of commonly studied adolescent marijuana use determinants in Italy. Continued efforts should be made to better explain both the risk and protective factors of marijuana use among Italian adolescents.

INTRODUCTION

Although a host of norms and regulations prohibit underage youth the use of substances, we know that the use of alcohol, tobacco, and marijuana are widespread among this population. In Italy the socio-cultural norms and policies regarding the use of psychoactive substances among adolescents varies greatly. While the use of certain substances such as alcohol are encouraged and even guided by the family during adolescence, others such as marijuana are strictly prohibited. Mmarijuana use is one of the first drugs that youths try after alcohol and tobacco (Ciairano, 2009 Bonino, & Miceli, 2008).

Indeed, The European School Survey Project on Alcohol and Other Drugs' (ESPAD) most recent report showed that the vast majority of 15–16 year-old European students in 35 member countries who had tried illicit drugs had used marijuana (Hibell, 2009). More worrisome is the fact that trend data from consecutive cross-sectional surveys in Europe have shown a general increase in the prevalence of marijuana use among adolescents (Hibell, 2009). The 2003 ESPAD survey reported a stable development for most countries (Hibell, Andersson, Bjarnasson, Ahlstöm, Balakireva, Kokkevi, & Morgan, 2004). In 2007 lifetime cannabis use was reported by 19% of the students (Hibell, 2009). Seven percent of all ESPAD students stated that they had used marijuana or hashish during the last 30 days. This corresponds to roughly one-third of the group reporting lifetime use (Hibell, 2009). Use of marijuana in the past 12 months was reported by 16% of the boys and 12% of the girls (14% of all students). Almost 9 in 10 students who had ever used marijuana had apparently done so during the past 12 months (Hibell, 2009).

In Italy the use of marijuana is slightly more frequent than in many other ESPAD countries (23% vs. 19% for the total sample) (Hibell, 2009). This rate is noteworthy considering that Italy has undertaken a moderate prohibitionist position against the use of marijuana in that it does not distinguish between the use of soft and hard drugs, which are both considered illegal.

It is also worth noting that Italy has been reported to have one of the highest proportions of high-risk users in Europe according to the Cannabis Abuse Screening Test (CAST) (Beck & Legleye, 2003), a questionnaire that is intended to screen for different aspects of harmful cannabis use by assessing the frequency of seemingly non-recreational use: smoking before midday and alone, memory disorders, being encouraged to reduce using cannabis, unsuccessful quit attempts and problems linked to cannabis consumption.

This cross-national assessment showed that Italy rated third out of seventeen participating countries in use before midday; fourth in use when being alone; third in problematic use patterns; and second in problems related to cannabis consumption (arguments, fights, accidents or bad results at school because of their use of cannabis). The survey assessment also evaluated the proportion of high-risk marijuana consumers related to the total sample of students. The highest rates were reported in Italy (3%), Monaco (3%), Czech Republic (4%) and Isle of Man (4%).

These reports evidence the great need to understand the types of determinants that are influencing the high prevalence rates of adolescent marijuana use in Italy, as well as the apparent problematic use behaviors that this population is exhibiting.

Referring to the etiology of youth substance use including marijuana there is extensive literature identifying and associating selected intrapersonal and environmental risk factors for substance use behaviors. Investigation efforts in underage substance use have focused on the young individual's intrapersonal characteristics, on their family life, and on their school experience (Hawkins, Catalano, & Miller, 1992; Zweig, Phillips, & Lindberg, 2002) to explain this phenomenon.

The intrapersonal risk factors that have been identified for youth substance use include depression (Deykin, Levy, & Wells, 1987) (Grant & Harford, 1995; Kumpulainen, 2002; Regier, Farmer, Rae, Locke, Keith, Goodwin, & Goodwin, 1990) (Gilman & Abraham, 2001), stress (Abrams & Niaura, 1987; Cooper, Russell, Skinner, Frone, & Mudar, 1992; Wills & Hirky, 1996), and hostility (Andersson, Magnusson, & Wennberg, 1997; Windle & Windle, 1995). Reviews have also suggested that trait dispositions such as sensation seeking and risk taking play roles in the development of substance use (Hawkins, Catalano, & Miller, 1992; Petraitis, Flay, & Miller, 1995): children are more likely to develop substance use disorders later on if they exhibit high levels of novelty-seeking behavior.

Risk factors from the adolescent's environment include parental characteristics such as the level of control that their parents have over their personal decisions and tolerance or approval of problem behavior. Other environmental risk factors include the academic performance of the youths and the substance use status of their friends. Affiliation with substance-using peers has been reported to encourage different aspects of substance use behaviors (onset, persistence, and intoxication) through various mechanisms, including social learning, peer group influence, modeling, and social facilitation (Sher et al, 2005; Engels, Hermans, van Baaren, Hollenstein, and Bot, 2009).

Nonetheless, it is worth noting that most studies investigating determinants of adolescent marijuana use fail to concentrate on marijuana use exclusively. There are a host of issues particular to the problem of adolescent marijuana use that may be beyond the scope of multi-substance use investigations that need to be addressed with greater detail and focus. The difficulties in analyzing common risk/protective factors associated with the use behaviors of multiple substances are not only that dependence and outcomes are characteristically different between substances, but that the risk/protective factors associated with transition behaviors may be different for every substance. Thus we risk missing important risk/protective factor nuances that may distinguish between use transition behaviors among different substances. Further, we know that those who become dependent on illicit drugs differ from those who become dependent on nicotine and alcohol in sex ratio, age, employment (Hughes, 2006). There are also marked differences between tobacco, alcohol and other drug use dependencies; marijuana dependence for example almost never causes adverse behavioral outcomes such as violence, suicide, risky sexual behaviors, child neglect, etc (Hughes, 2006) which may also influence escalation of use between different substances.

Furthermore, some of the more important adolescent substance determinants identified in the literature pertain to both the intrapersonal and environmental domains of youths' lives; however few studies looking at the influence of potential interpersonal determinants on adolescent substance use neglect to study the concomitant effects of environmental influences on adolescent substance use onset and continued use in single models of analysis.

The purpose of this investigation was to gain a better understanding of how particular adolescent substance use determinants that have been uncovered in distinct populations would predict the marijuana use behaviors of Italian adolescents one year later. For this reason we have considered a set of potential marijuana use determinants among the following domains: personal: (depression, stress, aggression, sensation seeking, and risk taking), family (strict family rule and parent approval of marijuana use), peer (peer approval of marijuana use and peer marijuana use) and school context (academic marks). Our goal was to investigate how these factors associated longitudinally with three marijuana use indicators: lifetime use, past six month use, and intoxication.

We know that relative social and psychological maladjustment tends to predate initiation of substance use onset and subsequent disorders such as intoxication (Shedler, 1990). Thus, we expected marijuana to be used as a compensatory coping strategy for dealing with emotional distress. That is we expected to find associations between depression, stress and marijuana use.

Given that several studies have shown strong relationships between substance use and aggression, and that some research supports a common bio-behavioral basis for the development of both (Weiner, 2001; Griffin, 2003), we expected to find associations between aggression and intoxication. Also Since sensation seeking and risk taking appear to be personal stable traits; we hypothesized the presence of an association with intoxication and past sic month use.

Considering both literature findings (Hartos & Power; Loukas & Prelow) and the great relevance of the Italian family in adolescent development (Bonino, Cattelino and Ciairano, 2006; Claes, 1998), we expected that stricter family rules would associate negatively with marijuana use. Likewise considering the prohibitionist position Italians have taken on marijuana use, we did not expect that parental approval would be related to adolescent marijuana use behaviors.

Several studies have emphasized the role of peers in influencing substance use (Deater-Deckard 2001; Sher et al, 2005). Closeness and intimacy become important features within adolescent friendships (Ciairano, Rabaglietti, Roggero, Bonino, & Beyers, 2007), thus we expected that higher levels of peer modeling, and approval of problem behavior would associate with greater marijuana use. Lastly, considering that general substance use has been associated with lower academic achievement and negative perceptions of school in as early as 6th grade students (Ellickson, Tucker, & Klein, 2001; Sobeck, Abbey, Agius, Clinton, & Harrison, 2000), we expected to observe a negative association between academic achievement and marijuana use.

We also assessed the effect of gender as a potential moderating effect between our study determinants and the selected indicators of marijuana use. Recent studies have shown that gender differences in important risk behaviors are beginning to disappear in current Italian society. A recent study looking at various adolescent risk behaviors among Italian youth found no gender differences in various substance use consumption behaviors (Ciairano, 2008 Bosma, 2005). This equalization of risk behaviors has been explained in part due to the fact that the role of young women in Italian society is rapidly evolving where they are currently experiencing new demands like pursuing higher educations and careers (Bonino, 2005, 2006). However differences still exist in the way girls are being brought up, especially in terms of housework responsibilities and freedom outside home (Bonino, 2005, 2006). The presence of these gender differences in the socialization processes of Italian boys and girls seems to continue to influence risk behavior determinants that the underlie processes of involvement in different kinds of risk behavior. For instance, girls are much more involved than boys in internalizing behavior (such as disturbed eating and depression) and boys have a greater involvement than girls in typically externalizing behaviors (such as aggression) (Ciairano, 2004; Ciairano, Kliewer, Bonino, Bosma, 2005).

This investigation's contribution to the field of youth marijuana use is that it will help us gain an increasingly refined understanding of the etiological factors that contribute to marijuana use onset and how these factors interrelate with one another to contribute to progression along the gamut of adolescent marijuana use involvement. A more detailed understanding of the factors that influence marijuana use initiation and consumption behavior can help guide prevention investigators in the field to focus on specific risk factors or combinations of risk and protective factors which may promote delays of marijuana use onset or curb progression to heavier use along different points of transition. Also of great importance is that this investigation contributed to our knowledge of Italian youth marijuana use behaviors; an area of investigation that is in great need of advancement for the development of prevention programs that take into account the determinants of Italian youth marijuana use.

METHODS

Procedure

Research was conducted in the Italian province of Turin which is situated in Northern Italy. A sample of public high schools stratified by school type was invited to participate. Students and parents were informed about the study and all agreed to participate providing written consent. Trained researchers administered the questionnaire at school without teachers being present. All sampled youth completed the questionnaires, although a number of students skipped some answers and thus list-wise procedures excluded them from the analyses.

Participants

The sample consisted of 324 youths (56% male) ranging in age from 15-20 (M = 17.29 yrs, SD = 1.61) living in northwest Italy. Nearly all (89.6%) of the parents were married and lived together. Half (50%) of the mothers and 86% of the fathers worked full-time; an additional 11% of the mothers worked part-time and 31% were housewives. A total of 6% of both fathers and mothers had a University degree. We included diverse types of secondary schools as schools that focused on high educational tracks (25.3%) and schools that focused on technical training (74.7%). A total of 4 schools were involved in this study: 1 vocational high school (6 classes with 130 total students), 1 lyceum high school (4 classes with 81 total students), and 2 technical high schools (7 classes with 113 total students). Of the total 324 students invited to participate at baseline 100% agreed to participate. A total of 22 students were lost at the one year follow up time point. Reasons for loss at follow up included absence from school and moving to different schools. Thus, after excluding students with missing data at follow-up, the number of students included in the models was 302.

Attrition Analyses

Attrition analysis was conducted by analyzing the least square mean differences in demographic and study variables of interest between those with complete follow up data and those participants who were lost at follow up. Mean scores of demographic variables and of our study variables of interest were not significantly different.

Overview of the Assessment Strategy

Measures used in this study were derived from the Italian version of the *Health Behavior Questionnaire* (Bonino, Cattelino, & Ciairano, 2006). The scales and composite measures of the questionnaire are all theoretically-derived and have been widely used over the past couple of decades (Jessor, Donovan, & Costa, 1991). Validity of the scales has been established across multiple studies and multiple populations (Jessor, Donovan, & Costa, 1992; Jessor, Turbin, Costa, Dong, Zhang, & Wang, 2003), including Italy (Ciairano, 2006; Molinengo, 2010).

Study Variables

Depression evaluated: to feel really down about things, to feel pretty hopeless about the future, to spend a lot of time worrying about little things, to feel depressed about life in general, to feel lonely (5 items). Cronbach's Alpha was .76 at baseline and .77 at follow-up.

Sensation seeking evaluated if the participants felt they were prepared to use drugs: to experiment new sensations, to prove that you are able to, to feel myself stronger, to share with friend something dangerous, to share with friend something exciting and new. Cronbach's Alpha was .77 at baseline and .80 at follow-up.

Stress was evaluated by asking participants rate how stressed they felt in social relations, in school, and in their family lives. Possible answers: no (1), a little (2), fairly (3), and a lot (4).

Aggression evaluated if during the past six months, how often the adolescent had: started a fight, hit someone, been in a fight, carried a weapon, had a serious fight at school (5 items). Cronbach's Alpha was .80 at baseline and .82 at follow-up.

Risk-taking evaluated during the past six months, how often the adolescents has: done something dangerous just for the thrill of it; dome some risky things because it was exciting; taken chances wit h one's safety when one was out at night because it was exciting (3 items) The possible answers to each question are: never (1), sometimes (2), often (3), always (4). Cronbach's Alpha was .80 at baseline and .82 at follow-up.

School marks evaluated the students past academic achievement as indicated by their last school marks.

Strict family rule evaluated how strict the rules are the adolescents had to follow : when and which television shows they can watch, letting family know where they're going, getting their homework done, dating with the partner, going to parties, being at home by a certain time at night, getting chores done around the house (8 items). Cronbach's Alpha was .71 at baseline and .76 at follow-up.

Parental approval of marijuana use evaluated the approval of parents about the involvement of the adolescents with marijuana use. The possible answers were: disapprove (1), neither disapprove nor approve (2), approve (3).

Friends' approval of marijuana use It evaluated the approval of friends about the involvement of the adolescents with marijuana use. The possible answers were: disapprove (1), neither disapprove nor approve (2), approve (3).

Peer marijuana use evaluated how many of their friends use marijuana? response answers ranged from none, some, most, all.

Life time marijuana use evaluated if they had ever tried marijuana. Response choices included no, never, yes, once; and yes, more than once.

Past six month use asked In the past six months, how many times have you smoked marijuana? response choices included: Never; Once; 2-3 times; 4-5 times; Once a month 5; 2-3 times a month; Once a week; 2-3 times a week; 4-5 times a week; Every day.

Intoxication evaluated if they had ever been high or stoned from using marijuana? response choices included: No, never; Yes, once; Yes, more than once; Yes, always

Also included in the analyses were the demographic variables of age, gender and highest level of parental education.

Analyses

The analysis included non-missing data from student respondents at two time points. They were performed on one year follow-up data. Because individuals were sampled within different school types, autocorrelation of respondents would violate the assumption of independence for ordinary least squares regression analyses, potentially shrinking standard errors and increasing type I error rates. Due to the clustering of students within schools and the possible intra-school correlation between students within the same school, a general linear mixed model was applied in the analysis. Mixed-model regression methods accommodate any degree of dependence present in the data by modeling it explicitly (Murray, 1998). Multilevel structure indicates that data to be analyzed were obtained from various levels, and these levels are nested within each other. PROC MIXED SAS Version 9.0 (SAS, 1999) was for the analysis of the dependent variables: lifetime use, past six month use, and intoxication.

We analyzed the 1 year follow up associations between the personal, family, peer, and school domain determinants and each of the three indications of adolescent marijuana use. In order to determine if differences existed between genders we explored its moderating effect on the relationships between selected determinants and indicators of tobacco use. All independent variables were tested in a single model in order to control for individual effects. Possible confounders adjusted for in the analyses included age, gender and highest level of parental education.

RESULTS

Characteristics of Participants

At baseline over 50% of both males and females indicated having some friends who smoked marijuana; approximately 20% indicated that most of their friends smoked marijuana. Regarding lifetime marijuana use, approximately 65% of the sample indicated never having smoked marijuana, while roughly 26% indicated having smoked more than once. Approximately 33% of the sample indicated never having been intoxicated by marijuana; and approximately 40% indicated having been intoxicated more than once.

Table 1. Summary of study variables by gender

N = 302		Male			Female			
		%	Mean	SD	%	Mean	SD	P
Age			16.76			16.97		NS
School type								
	High school	21.3			30.83			<.0001
	Technical	52.07			9.77			
	Professional	26.63			59.4			
Depression			2.03	0.63		2.51	0.65	<.0001
Aggression			1.28	0.45		1.11	0.35	0.0005
Sensation seeking			2.57	1.14		2.32	0.92	0.05
Stress			2.26	0.31		2.56	0.31	<.0001
Risk Taking			1.50	0.61		1.38	0.52	NS
School marks			6.36	0.61		6.34	0.61	NS
Strict family rule			2.35	0.55		2.43	0.48	NS
Parent approval of problem behavior			1.33	0.31		1.33	0.31	NS
Peer approval of problem behavior			2.09	0.48		2.13	0.55	NS
Peer marijuana use								NS
	None	22.16			20.30			
	Some	55.09			51.13			
	Most	19.16			24.81			
	All	3.59			3.76			
Lifetime marijuana use								NS
	No, never	65.27			64.66			
	Yes, once	8.38			8.27			
	Yes, more than once	26.35			27.07			
Past six month marijuana use Frequency								NS
	Never	12.07			14.89			
	Once	29.31			23.40			
	2-3 times	24.14			8.51			
	4-5 times	1.72			6.38			
	Once a month	8.62			4.26			
	2-3 times a month	6.90			12.77			
	Once a week	5.17			4.26			
	2-3 times a week	3.45			8.51			
	4-5 times a week	5.17			6.38			
	Every day	3.45			10.64			
Marijuana use Intoxication	No, never	34.48			32.61			NS
	Yes, once	18.97			15.22			
	Yes, more than once	37.93			41.30			
	Yes, always	8.62			10.87			

Table 2. Italian Adolescent Marijuana Determinants by Marijuan a Involvement, 1 year follow up Analysis

N = 302***		Beta Estimates*								
		Lifetime use			Past 6 mo use freq			6 mo intoxication frequency		
Domain	Effect**	β	SE	P	β	SE	P	β	SE	P
	Baseline Marijuana use	0.653	0.058	<.0001	0.518	0.120	<.0001	0.304	0.105	0.0051
	Depression	-0.238	0.114	0.0292	2.668	0.878	0.0040	-0.286	0.311	0.3703
	Aggression	-0.081	0.134	0.3458	1.687	1.217	0.2909	-0.518	0.434	0.2750
Personal	Stress	0.145	0.110	0.0328	-0.782	0.851	0.2656	0.766	0.306	0.0077
	Sensation seeking	-0.010	0.046	0.0088	0.710	0.387	0.1945	-0.063	0.141	0.7618
	Risk taking	0.102	0.097	0.2658	-0.056	0.661	0.6065	-0.245	0.239	0.9618
Academic	School marks	-0.110	0.089	0.2057	-0.804	0.789	0.2681	-0.306	0.282	0.1329
	Strict family rules	-0.322	0.101	0.0048	-1.545	0.658	0.0224	-0.359	0.238	0.0345
Family	Parent approval of marijuana use	0.040	0.174	0.0752	0.282	1.112	0.8245	0.374	0.403	0.3490
Peer	Peer approval of marijuana use	0.084	0.125	0.9855	-0.398	1.096	0.1513	-0.026	0.399	0.3623
	Peer marijuana use	0.073	0.087	0.3512	0.860	0.593	0.0651	0.011	0.210	0.6992
	Age	-0.059	0.032	0.0683	-0.466	0.214	0.0332	-0.123	0.077	0.1175
Demographics	Gender	-1.734	1.182	0.2803	5.675	9.234	0.6014	0.222	3.353	0.9532
	Parent education	0.026	0.023	0.2626	0.090	0.14	0.5418	0.029	0.052	0.5687
Interactions	Depression*Gender	0.098	0.172	0.5683	-1.356	1.298	0.2999	0.142	0.466	0.7609
	Aggression*Gender	-0.060	0.232	0.7943	-1.664	1.523	0.2788	0.406	0.547	0.4611
	Stress*Gender	0.076	0.170	0.6525	0.193	1.126	0.8641	-0.326	0.411	0.4296
	Sensation seeking*Gender	0.235	0.082	0.0045	-0.562	0.652	0.3920	0.199	0.237	0.4052
	Risk taking*Gender	-0.021	0.162	0.8928	-0.427	1.045	0.6840	0.472	0.395	0.2365
	School marks*Gender	0.049	0.134	0.7120	0.335	1.026	0.7446	-0.000	0.371	0.9982
	Strict family rules*Gender	0.165	0.167	0.3239	0.236	1.197	0.8439	-0.278	0.448	0.5373
	Parent approval of marijuana use*Gender	0.390	0.260	0.1340	-0.958	1.744	0.5846	-0.148	0.634	0.8156
	Peer approval of marijuana use*Gender	-0.172	0.174	0.3245	-1.263	1.445	0.3852	-0.429	0.531	0.4219
	Peer marijuana use*Gender	-0.015	0.128	0.9055	0.223	0.943	0.8136	0.124	0.382	0.7454

* Adjusted for age, grade and highest level of parental education.

** Variables from each domain were tested in a single model in order to control for individual effects.

*** Due to the clustering of students within schools a mixed model was applied in the analysis with school type as the clustering variable.

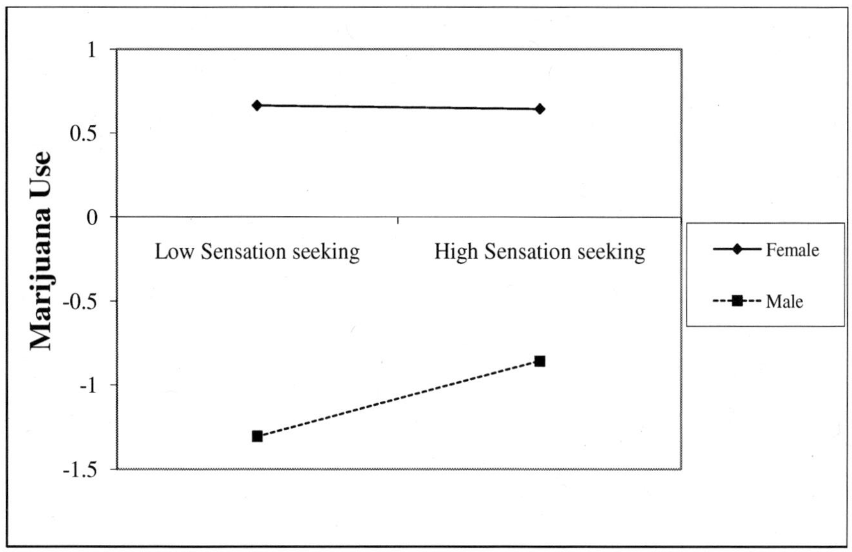

Figure 1. Gender moderation analysis between lifetime marijuana use and sensation seeking.

Statistically significant difference was found between genders. Females reported significantly higher mean levels of depression ($\chi = 2.51$ vs. $\chi = 2.03$, $p < .0001$), and total stress ($\chi = 2.56$ vs. $\chi = 2.26$, $p < .0001$). Males on the other hand reported higher levels of aggression ($\chi = 1.28$ vs. $\chi = 1.11$, $p < .0001$), and higher levels of sensation seeking ($\chi = 2.57$ vs. $\chi = 2.32$, $p = .05$).

Relationships among Marijuana Use and Study Determinants

Lifetime Marijuana Use

One year follow up analyses revealed that higher indications of depression at baseline were negatively associated with lifetime marijuana use at 1 year follow up ($\beta = -0.24$, $p = 0.03$). This indicates that higher indications of depression at baseline were associated with lower indications of marijuana use at one year follow up. Similarly higher indications of sensation seeking at baseline were negatively associated with lifetime marijuana use at 1 year follow up ($\beta = -0.010$, $p = 0.008$). On the other hand higher indications of stress at baseline were associated with higher indications of lifetime marijuana use at follow up ($\beta = 0.14$, $p = 0.03$). Lastly, a greater perception of strict family rules at baseline was associated with lower indications of lifetime marijuana use at 1 year follow up ($\beta = -0.32$, $p = 0.005$). Moderation analyses revealed a significant gender interaction between the association of sensation seeking and lifetime marijuana use ($\beta = 0.23$, $p = 0.004$) indicating that the relationship between sensation seeking and lifetime marijuana use varied by gender (see figure 1).

Past Six Month Use Frequency

Opposite to our results with lifetime marijuana use, when looking at past six month use frequency results showed that higher indications of depression at baseline were associated with greater indications of marijuana use in the past six months ($\beta = 2.66$, $p = 0.004$). As with lifetime marijuana use a greater perception of strict family rules at baseline was associated with lower indications of past six month marijuana use frequency at 1 year follow up ($\beta = -1.54$, $p = 0.02$). Results also showed that older participants indicated lower past six month use frequency ($\beta = -0.46$, $p = 0.03$).

Intoxication

Similar to our findings with lifetime marijuana use a greater perception of stress at baseline was associated with higher indications of marijuana use intoxication at 1 year follow up ($\beta = 0.76$, $p = 0.007$). As with each other dependent variable, results showed that a greater perception of strict family rules at baseline was associated with lower indications of marijuana use intoxication at 1 year follow up ($\beta = -0.35$, $p = 0.03$).

CONCLUSION

The purpose of this investigation was to gain a better understanding of the marijuana use determinants of Italian adolescents. We investigated the one year longitudinal effects of our samples' personal (depression, stress, aggression, sensation seeking, and risk taking), family (strict family rule and parent approval of marijuana use), peer (peer approval of marijuana use and peer marijuana use) and school (academic marks) domains on three marijuana use indicators: lifetime use, past six month use frequency, and intoxication.

While such determinants have been previously investigated in association to general adolescent substance use behaviors, few investigations have concentrated on the effects that these determinants have on adolescent marijuana use exclusively. One goal of this investigation was to see how these determinants predicted the marijuana use behaviors of a sample of Italian adolescents, a population that is among the highest in Europe for high-risk marijuana consumption (Hibell, 2009). Another goal of this investigation was to study the effect of our selected determinants in a single statistical model in order to study how predictors from various life domains affected adolescent marijuana use concomitantly. Lastly we investigated if gender differences existed among these associations

With respect to personal domain determinants, this paper showed that higher indications of depression at baseline were associated with lower indications of marijuana use at one year follow up. While several studies have shown strong associations between depression and substance use, these associations may be more present when considering heavier modes of substance use and not indications of experimentation as was our indicator of lifetime marijuana use. Indeed this was somewhat confirmed when we analyzed the association between past six month use frequency as results showed that higher indications of depression at baseline were associated with greater indications of frequency of marijuana use in the past six months. These results may point to the fact that heavier modes of marijuana use may represent a compensatory coping strategy for depression among Italian adolescents, but that depression may not be an important determining factor for marijuana use onset. In the case of our study, we need to underline that our participants did not belong to any kind of populations at clinical risk for depression or other kinds of psychological discomfort: they were normative developing adolescents who regularly attended high school. Further studies must further explore this issue possibly with clinical samples of depression and with longer longitudinal studies that could capture the nuances of marijuana use onset and transition use behaviors among adolescent.

Our results showed that marijuana use may indeed be utilized as a coping strategy for feelings of stress in our population as greater indications of lifetime marijuana use and higher indications of marijuana use intoxication at 1 year follow up were associated with greater indications of stress. Further studies should take care to investigate why marijuana is being selected as a coping strategy. One possible answer lies on the fact that, as the latest ESPAD report shows, a total of one-third of the students in the ESPAD countries reported finding marijuana readily available (Hibell, 2009). If this is indeed the case then studies such as this one can serve to inform policy makers and prevention scientists as to the uses that adolescents are finding in such a widely available drug. Efforts should be directed at educating adolescents on alternative stress coping strategies.

As indicated earlier, reviews have suggested that trait dispositions such as sensation seeking and risk taking play roles in the development of substance use (Hawkins, Catalano, & Miller, 1992; Petraitis, Flay, & Miller, 1995). However other investigators have reported mixed findings for trait dispositions such as sensation seeking (Simon, 1994). Our results showed that higher indications of sensation seeking at baseline were negatively associated with lifetime marijuana use at 1 year follow up and that the relationship between sensation seeking and lifetime marijuana use varied by gender. This finding confirms the reports of Martin, Kelly, Rayens, Brogli, Brenzel, Smith, Omar (Martin, 2002) which found that sensation seeking was positively associated with pubertal development, even when controlling for age, and that sensation seeking mediated the relationship of pubertal development and drug use in both boys and girls. The lack of association between sensation seeking and lifetime marijuana use may be due to the fact that marijuana acts as a depressor to the central nervous system thus depriving the individual from seeking novel sensations.

As for our environmental domains, it seems that parenting was the most effective protective factor for every marijuana use behavior we investigated. A greater perception of strict family rules was associated with lower indications of lifetime marijuana use, past six month use frequency and with marijuana intoxication. This finding can serve to inform prevention efforts which should take into account the strong influence that parenting has on delay of marijuana use experimentation onset and heavier modes of use.

This study has several limitations as the presence of just two waves, and the small sample size. Due to these limitations we were unable to distinguish among different marijuana use trajectories (Schulenberg, Maggs, 2002). A study of this type may also benefit of a longer period of study which could allow us to identify how these associations are present throughout multiple waves. This would allow us to track how specific determinants affect not only marijuana use onset but later stages such as maintenance and subsequent heavier usage. This study represents a first attempt to uncover the marijuana use determinants of Italian adolescents. While not every important explaining factor has been studied here we have attempted to look at the effects of commonly studied adolescent marijuana use determinants in Italy. Continued efforts should be made in order to better explain both the risk and protective factors of marijuana use among Italian adolescents.

REFERENCES

Abrams, D. B., & Niaura, R. S. (1987). Social learning theory. In H. T. Blane & K. E. Leonard (Eds.), *Psychological theories of drinking and alcoholism* (pp. 131–178). New York: Guilford.

Andersson, T., Magnusson, D., & Wennberg, P. (1997). Early aggressiveness and hyperactivity as indicators of adult alcohol problems and criminality: a prospective longitudinal study of male subjects. *Studies on Crime and Crime Prevention*, *6*, 7-20.

Beck, F., & Legleye, S. (2003). *Drogues et adolescents. Usages de drogues et contextes d'usage entre 17 et 19 ans, évolutions récentes, ESCAPAD (2002)*. Paris: OFDT.

Bonino, S., Cattelino, E., & Ciairano, S. (2006). Italy. In J. J. Arnett (Ed.), *International Encyclopedia of Adolescence* (Vol. 2, pp. 510-523). New York-London: Routledge.

Bonino, S., Cattelino, E., & Ciairano, S. (2005). *Adolescents and risk. Behaviors, functions and protective factors*. New York: Springer Verlag.

Bonino, S., Cattelino, E., & Ciairano, S. (2006). Italy. In J. J. Arnett (Ed.), *International Encyclopedia of Adolescence* (pp. 510-523). London & New York: Routledge.

Ciairano, S., Kliewer, W., Bonino, S., & Bosma H. (2008). Parenting and Adolescent Well-Being in Two European Countries. *Adolescence*, *43*, 99-117.

Ciairano, S., Molinengo, G., Bonino, S., Miceli, R., van Schuur, W. (2009). Age of initiation with different substances and relationships with resources and vulnerabilities: A cross-national study. *European Journal of Developmental Psychology*, *6*(6), 666-684.

Ciairano, S., van Schuur, W., Molinengo, G., Bonino, S., Miceli, R. (2006). The use of psychoactive substances among Dutch and Italian adolescents: The contribution of personal and relational resources and vulnerabilities. *European Journal of Developmental Psychology*, *3*(4), 321 - 337.

Cooper, M. L., Russell, M., Skinner, J. B., Frone, M. R., & Mudar, P. (1992). Stress and alcohol use: Moderating effects of gender, coping and alcohol expectancies. *Journal of Abnormal Psychology*, *101*, 139–152.

Deykin, E. Y., Levy, J. C., & Wells, V. (1987). Adolescent depression, alcohol and drug abuse. *American Journal of Public Health*, *77*, 178–182.

Ellickson, P. L., Tucker, J. S., & Klein, D. J. (2001). High-risk behaviors associated with early smoking: Results from a 5-year follow-up. *Journal of Adolescent Health*, *28*(6), 465–473.

Gilman, S. E., & Abraham, H. D. (2001). A longitudinal study of the order of onset of alcohol dependence and major depression. *Drug & Alcohol Dependence*, *63*, 277-286.

Grant, B. F., & Harford, T. C. (1995). Comorbidity between DSM-IV alcohol use disorders depression: results of a national survey and major depression: results of a national survey. *Drug and Alcohol Dependence*, *39*, 197-206.

Hartos, J. L., & Power, T. G. (2000). Relations Among Single Mothers' Awareness of Their Adolescents' Stressors, Maternal Monitoring, Mother-Adolescent Communication, and Adolescent Adjustment. *Journal of Adolescent Research*, *15*(5), 546-563.

Hawkins, J. D., Catalano, J. F., & Miller, J. Y. (1992). Risk and Protective Factors for Alcohol and other Drug Problems in Adolescence and Early Adulthood: Implications for Substance Abuse Prevention. *Psychological Bulletin*, *112*, 64-105.

Hibell, B., Andersson, B., Bjarnasson, T., Ahlstöm, S., Balakireva, O., Kokkevi, A., & Morgan, M. (2004). *The ESPAD Report 2003. Alcohol and Other Drug Use Among Students in 35 European Countries*: The Swedish Council for Information on Alcohol and Other Drugs (CAN) and The Council of Europe, Co-operation Group to Combat Drug Abuse and Illicit Trafficing in Drugs (Pompidou Group).

Hibell, B., Guttormsson, U., Ahlström, S., Balakireva, O., Bjarnason T., Kokkevi A., Kraus, L. (2009). *The ESPAD Report 2007. Alcohol and Other Drug Use Among Students in 35 European Countries.* Stockholm, Sweden: The Swedish Council for Information on Alcohol and Other Drugs.

Hughes, J. R. (2006). Should criteria for drug dependence differ across drugs? *Addiction*, *101*(s1), 134–141.

Jessor, R., Donovan, J. E., & Costa, F. M. (1991). *Beyond adolescence - Problem behavior and young adult development.* New York: Cambridge University Press.

Jessor, R., Donovan, J. E., & Costa, F. M. (1992). *Health behavior Questionnaire. High School form.* Boulder, CO: Institute of Behavioral Science, University of Colorado Boulder.

Jessor, R., Turbin, M. S., Costa, F. M., Dong, Q., Zhang, H., & Wang, C. (2003). Adolescent Problem Behavior in China and the United States: A Cross-National Study of Psychosocial Protective factors. *Journal of Research on Adolescence*, *13*(1), 329-360.

Kumpulainen, K. (2002). Depressive symptoms at the age of 12 years and future heavy alcohol use. *Addictive Behaviors*, *27*, 425–436.

Loukas, A., & Prelow, H. M. (2004). Externalizing and Internalizing Problems in Low-Income Latino Early Adolescents: Risk, Resource, and Protective Factors. *Journal of Early Adolescence*, *24*(3), 250-273.

Martin, A. C., Kelly, H., Rayens, K.M., Brogli, R.B., Brenzel, A., Smith, W.J., Omar, R.A. . (2002). Sensation seeking, puberty, and nicotine, alcohol, and marijuana use in adolescence. *Journal of the American Academy of Child & Adolescent Psychiatry*, *41*, 1495-1502.

Molinengo, G., Testa, S. (2010). Analysis of the Psychometric Properties of an Assessment Tool for Deviant Behavior in Adolescence. *European Journal of Psychological Assessment*, *26*(2), 108-115.

Murray, D. M. (1998). *Design and Analysis of Group-Randomized Trials*. New York, NY: Oxford Univ. Press.

Regier, M. E., Farmer, D. S., Rae, B. Z., Locke, S. J., Keith, L. L., Goodwin, J., & Goodwin, F. K. (1990). Comorbidity of mental disorders with alcohol and other drug abuse. *JAMA*, *264*, 2511–2518.

SAS. (1999). SAS system for Windows software (Version release 8). NC: SAS Institute.

Shedler, J., Block, J. (1990). Adolescent Drug Use and Psychological Health: A longitudinal Inquiry. *American Psychologist*, *45*(5), 612-630.

Simon, T. R., Stacy, A.W., Sussman, S., Dent, C.W. . (1994). Sensation seeking and drug use among high risk Latino and Anglo adolescents. *Personality and Individual Differences*, *17*(5), 665-672.

Sobeck, J., Abbey, A., Agius, E., Clinton, M., & Harrison, K. (2000). Predicting early adolescent substance use: Do risk factors differ depending on age of onset? *Journal of Substance Abuse*, *11*(1), 89–102.

Wills, T. A., & Hirky, E. (Eds.). (1996). *Coping and substance abuse: A theoretical model and review of the evidence*. New York: Wiley.

Windle, R. C., & Windle, M. (1995). Longitudinal patterns of physical aggression: associations with adult social, psychiatric, and personality functioning and testosterone levels. *Developmental Psychology*, *7*, 563-585.

Zweig, J. M., Phillips, S. D., & Lindberg, L. D. (2002). Predicting Adolescent Profiles of Risk: Looking Beyond Demographics. *Journal of Adolescent Health*, *31*(4), 343-353.

In: Marijuana: Uses, Effects and the Law
Editor: Andrea S. Rojas
ISBN 978-1-61209-206-5

Chapter 7

RECREATIONAL MARIJUANA USE IN A BARIATRIC CLINIC POPULATION*

***Valerie Taylor*†,1 *and Arya Sharma*2**

[1]Mood Disorders Program, Centre for Mountain Health Services, St. Josephs's Healthcare, Hamilton, Ontario, Canada
[2]McMaster University, Ontario, Canada

ABSTRACT

Background: Use of marijuana for both medicinal and recreational purposes has been linked to the stimulation of appetite and weight gain. Anecdotal observation of patients in a bariatric clinic indicated that this population engaged in marijuana use, despite their problems with weight management. We conducted a chart review to see elucidate the marijuana use patterns in a bariatric population.

Methods: A retrospective chart review was done on 20 patients. Marijuana use was identified, as well as the use of cigarettes, alcohol and other illegal drugs, as well as age of obesity onset.

---

* A version of this chapter was also published in *New Research on Morbid Obesity,* edited by Wilma V. Parsons and Carolyn M. Taylor, published by Nova Science Publishers, Inc. It was for appropriate modifications in an effort to encourage wider dissemination of research.

† Correspondence should be addressed: D104-F, L8N 3K7, Fax: 905 575 6029; E-mail:taylorv@mcmaster.ca

Results: 25% of the patients used marijuana, which is higher that usage patterns for the general population (8.7%). Marijuana was not associated with use of other substances, or with age of onset of obesity.

Interpretation: We found a pattern of increased marijuana use in patients in a bariatric clinic. Further research is needed to better understand the nature of this finding and how it contributes to behavioral and pharmacological treatments of obesity.

Keywords: marijuana, obesity

Both the medicinal and recreational use of cannabis sativa (principal psychotropic component: Δ9-tetrahydrocannabinol) has been widely reported to result in the onset of a ravenous appetite and increased eating behavior ("the munchies"). Indeed, recreational use of marijuana has been shown to increase caloric intake and body weight [1] and medicinal use of marijuana has been evaluated as an appetite stimulant in cancer cachexia [2]. The most commonly reported reason for medicinal marijuana use in a recent study among a HIV population in Ontario, Canada, was appetite stimulation and weight gain [3]. These effects are believed to be mediated through activation of the CB_1 cannabinoid receptor [4]. Anecdotal observation that some patients with morbid obesity report regular marijuana use prompted us to systematically screen 20 consecutive patients with morbid obesity (BMI>40kg/m^2) who were referred for psychiatric assessment from a tertiary care bariatric clinic. (Table 1). History of marijuana use was elicited during the psychiatric interview from all patients. In morbidly obese patients referred for psychiatric assessment, the point prevalence of marijuana use was 25% This proportion of marijuana use is around 2.5 times higher than numbers found for marijuana use in the general Ontario population where 6.8% of adults above the age of 18 reported recreational use and 1.9% of respondents reported use of marijuana for medical purposes [5].

Since marijuana stimulates appetite and increases body weight[6], the high proportion of cannabis use in this population of bariatric clinic patients is especially relevant. The exact mechanisms behind these phenomenon have not been clearly elucidated as work with the cannabinoid system is new and the first receptor for Δ^9-THC was not fully characterized[7] until 1990. It has been suggested that the cannabinoid type 1(CB_1) receptor and its endogenous ligands, the endocannabinoids, are involved in controlling energy balance. The endocannabinoid system affects food intake via both central and peripheral mechanisms, and may also stimulate lipogenesis and fat accumulation [8]. It has also been suggested that the stimulation of CB_1 receptors may enhance food palatability [9].

Table 1. Marijuana use in patients attending a bariatric

	Marijuana use	No marijuana use
Female	3 (60%)	9 (60%)
	2 (40%)	6 (40%)
Obesity Onset		
Childhood (<10 y)	1 (20%)	5 (33.3%)
Adolescence (10–19 y)	3 (60%)	7 (46.6%)
Adult (>19 y)	1 (20%)	3 (20%)
Alcohol use*	5 (100%)	5 (33.3%)
Cigarette use	1 (20%)	4 (26.6%)

* Alcohol use did not exceed 1-2 drinks a week.

To our knowledge, cannabis use in a bariatric population has never been specifically examined, but extrapolating from work done on cannabis use in the community, it appears the vulnerabilities that may contribute to use, abuse and even dependence are clearly prevalent in this population. One contributing factor may be via mediators of physical health. The therapeutic possibilities of cannabis are currently being widely explored and a recent metaanalysis indicated that cannabinoids may be useful for conditions that currently lack effective treatment [10].

The use of cannabis for medical purposes is still controversial but despite the fact that most evidence supporting its use is anecdotal, cannabis has been used medicinally for a variety of conditions including chronic pain, menstrual cramps, migraine, narcotic addiction, stress and sleeping difficulties [11].

Many of these physical complaints are elevated in the bariatric population. With regard to sleep problems for example, obesity, especially when associated with an upper body distribution, is considered a major risk factor for obstructive sleep apnea (OSA). The estimates of prevalence of OSA in severely obese adults vary from 42–48% in men and 8–38% in women [12, 13]. Weight is also associated with co-morbid disability, depression, and reduced quality of life for physical function in chronic pain patients[14]. While exactly how excess weight can cause or contribute to pain has not been thoroughly studied, it is known that people who are overweight often are at greater risk for back pain, joint pain and muscle strain than those who are not obese [15]. The physical co-morbidity that is associated with obesity of physical illness may result in an increased need for bariatric patients to use coping strategies that include cannabis use.

The treatment of physical co-morbidity is not the only medicinal use of cannabis, and cannabis use is also related to several psychiatric disorders such as anxiety, depression, cognitive impairment, and psychosis. Clinical studies have reported that rates of depression are elevated among those seeking treatment for cannabis dependence [16] and, conversely, that rates of cannabis use are elevated among those seeking treatment for depression [17]. Cannabis use has also been linked to increases in anxiety disorders [18], and especially to symptoms of agoraphobia [19]. The co-morbidities between cannabis use and mental health problems may reflect process whereby depression and other mental health problems heighten the risk of substance use. The self-medication hypothesis posits that substance use may develop in response to attempts to ameleoriate aversive experiences associated with mental health problems [20]. Since substantial psychopathology exists in morbidly obese individuals [21], they have developing vulnerabilities predisposing to both cannabis use and an axis I psychiatry diagnosis. Cannabis use is also seen more frequently in populations that experience alienation from society [22] and given the diminished social integration, and stigmatization that some individuals with morbid obesity experience, this type of isolation is becoming more common in that group [23].

The link between psychiatric illness and the use of cannabis may also be related to difficulties that stem to back to childhood and early adolescence. Obesity has been shown significantly related to depression among 15- and 17-year-olds [24], with feeling of shame and experiences of being degraded or ridiculed by others often accounting for the association. Substance use in adolescents is also associated with well-documented risk factors such as peer group pressure and low self-esteem [25], so for a subgroup struggling with weight problems who are desperate to fit in, cannabis use may provide both a way to be accepted by a critical peer group and a means of self-medication against emotional problems. Cannabis initiation, as opposed to tobacco or alcohol, has also been shown to be significantly more prevalent among adolescents who are experiencing symptoms of depression prior to substance use [26]. This then places clinically obese adolescents, who have been shown to have higher rates of depressive symptomatology than non-clinical obese adolescents [27], at high risk of initiating a pattern of use that is then continued into adulthood.

Neurobiological explanations have also been put forward to explain the increased use of marijuana in certain at risk populations and these theories may also contribute to the increased drug usage seen in our bariatric population. Problems with impulsivity have been observed both in individuals with addictions (cocaine, marijuana, alcohol) as well as in individuals with Bulimia Nervosa, Binge Eating Disorder and those who eat in response to negative affect [28]. These patterns of disordered eating are more prevalent among overweight and obese persons than among those of normal weight [29] and may represent a problem with impulse control that predisposes to increased substance use. Interestingly, both pathological eating and drug addiction have been linked by a common attribution to aberrations in serotonin [30].

Another important neurobiological link may be at the level of the CB_1 receptor and cannabinoid regulation. During the past several years, cannabinoid biology has witnessed marked advances and we now have a better understanding of how the system works. The cannabinoid receptors are the biological targets for endogenous endocannabinoids such as N-arachidonyl ethanolamine (AEA). Prolonged activation of cannabinoid receptors observed after long-term exposure to synthetic or plant-derived cannabinoids leads to increased levels of AEA formation in areas of the brain such as the limbic forebrain [31]. This is relevant since animal studies indicate that the endocannabinoid system is important in stimulating food intake and when over stimulated contributes to hyperphagia, exaggerated fat accumulation and dyslipidemia. Such hyperactivity has been related to an increased availability of polyunsaturated fatty acid precursors for endocannabinoid biosynthesis caused by high-fat diets in obese patients, but this sustained hyperactivity of the endocannabinoid system may also explain weight gain associated with marijuana use [32]. Overweight and obesity in humans have also been shown recently to be associated with a potential genetic malfunctioning of one of the endocannabinoid degrading enzymes, further substantiating the hypothesis of a hyperactive endocannabinoid system as a possible cause of obesity [33].

The association between obesity and marijuana use is also highlighted by the proposed pharmacological treatment of both these conditions. A class of CB_1 selective endocannabinoid receptor antagonists are being developed for the treatment of obesity and show promise in helping control feelings of satiety. These drugs work by blocking endogenous cannabinoid binding to neuronal CB_1 receptors. Obesity treatment is not the only area that this drug class is being tested in and they have also shown promise in laboratory animals as a treatment of substance abuse [34, 35]. To our knowledge CB_1 antagonists have not been tested on cannabis reinforcing effects in humans but they have been effective in reducing drug-seeking behaviors in an animal analogue of relapse behaviors in human addicts [36]. The concept that one class of medication can be used to treat both difficulties in weight regulation secondary to increased food consumption, as well as addictive behaviors related to substance use imply that a shared vulnerability to problems in both areas may co-exist in some people.

This study is limited by its small sample size and lack of rigor quantifying the amount of marijuana use. It does indicate that further study is needed regarding co-morbid addictions in patients seeking treatment for obesity. Individuals suffering from obesity are at higher risk of physical health problems that the general population and this adverse outcome is exacerbated by the co-morbid use of marijuana. The reasons behind the elevated use of marijuana in this population are complex and encompass both biological vulnerabilities and reactions to societal pressures. The ability of newer treatment approaches to combat both issues is intriguing but it still does not fully address the factors that lead to substance use. It is important that substance use be screen for appropriately in this population and that appropriate resources are utilized in the management of substance use. If not, it will be very difficult to achieve satisfactory control of obesity.

REFERENCES

[1] Greenberg I, Kuehnle J, Mendelson JH, Bernstein JG. Effects of marihuana use on body weight and caloric intake in humans. *Psychopharmacology* (Berl*)* 1976 August 26;49(1):79-84.

[2] Hall W, Christie M, Currow D. Cannabinoids and cancer: causation, remediation, and palliation. *Lancet Oncol.* 2005 January;6(1):35-42.

[3] Furler MD, Einarson TR, Millson M, Walmsley S, Bendayan R. Medicinal and recreational marijuana use by patients infected with HIV. *AIDS Patient Care STDS* 2004 April;18(4):215-28.

[4] Vickers SP, Kennett GA. Cannabinoids and the regulation of ingestive behaviour. *Curr. Drug Targets* 2005 March;6(2):215-23.

[5] Ogborne AC, Smart RG, Adlaf EM. Self-reported medical use of marijuana: a survey of the general population. *CMAJ* 2000 June 13;162(12):1685-6.

[6] Kirkham TC. Endocannabinoids in the regulation of appetite and body weight. *Behav. Pharmacol.* 2005 September;16(5-6):297-313.

[7] Matsuda LA, Lolait SJ, Brownstein MJ, Young AC, Bonner TI. Structure of a cannabinoid receptor and functional expression of the cloned cDNA. *Nature* 1990 August 9;346(6284):561-4.
[8] Di M, V, Matias I. Endocannabinoid control of food intake and energy balance. *Nat. Neurosci.* 2005 May;8(5):585-9.
[9] Higgs S, Williams CM, Kirkham TC. Cannabinoid influences on palatability: microstructural analysis of sucrose drinking after delta(9)-tetrahydrocannabinol, anandamide, 2-arachidonoyl glycerol and SR141716. *Psychopharmacology* (Berl) 2003 February;165(4):370-7.
[10] Corey S. Recent developments in the therapeutic potential of cannabinoids. P R Health Sci J 2005 March;24(1):19-26.
[11] Ogborne AC, Smart RG, Weber T, Birchmore-Timney C. Who is using cannabis as a medicine and why: an exploratory study. *J. Psychoactive Drugs* 2000 October;32(4):435-43.
[12] Kyzer S, Charuzi I. Obstructive sleep apnea in the obese. *World J. Surg.* 1998 September;22(9):998-1001.
[13] Young T, Palta M, Dempsey J, Skatrud J, Weber S, Badr S. The occurrence of sleep-disordered breathing among middle-aged adults. *N. Engl. J. Med.* 1993 April 29;328(17):1230-5.
[14] Marcus DA. Obesity and the impact of chronic pain. *Clin. J. Pain* 2004 May;20(3):186-91.
[15] American Obesity Association. Health effects of obesity AOA Fact Sheets. http://www obesity org/subs/fastfacts/HealthEffects shtm*l* 2005.
[16] Aharonovich E, Nguyen HT, Nunes EV. Anger and depressive states among treatment-seeking drug abusers: testing the psychopharmacological specificity hypothesis *Am. J. Addict.* 2001;10 (4):327-34.
[17] Muser K, Yamold P, Belback A. Diagnostic and demographic correlates of substance abuse in schizophrenia and major affective disorder. *Acta Psychiatr. Scand* 1992;85:48-55.
[18] Agosti V, Nunes E, Levin F. Rates of psychiatric comorbidity among U.S. residents with lifetime cannabis dependence. *Am. J. Drug Alcohol. Abuse* 2002 November;28(4):643-52.
[19] Tournier M, Sorbara F, Gindre C, Swendsen JD, Verdoux H. Cannabis use and anxiety in daily life: a naturalistic investigation in a non-clinical population. *Psychiatry Res.* 2003 May 1;118(1):1-8.
[20] Khantzian EJ. The self-medication hypothesis of substance use disorders: a reconsideration and recent applications. *Harv. Rev. Psychiatry* 1997 January;4(5):231-44.

[21] Black DW, Goldstein RB, Mason EE. Prevalence of mental disorder in 88 morbidly obese bariatric clinic patients. *Am. J. Psychiatry* 1992 February;149(2):227-34.

[22] Sieber MF, Angst J. Alcohol, tobacco and cannabis: 12-year longitudinal associations with antecedent social context and personality. Drug Alcohol Depend 1990 June;25(3):281-92.

[23] Lissner L. Causes, diagnosis and risks of obesity. Pharmacoeconomics 1994;5(Suppl 1):8-17.

[24] Sjoberg RL, Nilsson KW, Leppert J. Obesity, shame, and depression in school-aged children: a population-based study. *Pediatrics* 2005 September; 116(3): e389-e392.

[25] von SK, Lieb R, Pfister H, Hofler M, Wittchen HU. What predicts incident use of cannabis and progression to abuse and dependence? A 4-year prospective examination of risk factors in a community sample of adolescents and young adults. *Drug Alcohol* Depend 2002 September 1;68(1):49-64.

[26] Libby AM, Orton HD, Stover SK, Riggs PD. What came first, major depression or substance use disorder? Clinical characteristics and substance use comparing teens in a treatment cohort. *Addict. Behav.* 2005 October;30(9):1649-62.

[27] Erermis S, Cetin N, Tamar M, Bukusoglu N, Akdeniz F, Goksen D. Is obesity a risk factor for psychopathology among adolescents? *Pediatr. Int.* 2004 June;46(3):296-301.

[28] Nasser JA, Gluck ME, Geliebter A. Impulsivity and test meal intake in obese binge eating women. *Appetite* 2004 December;43(3):303-7.

[29] Allison KC, Stunkard AJ. Obesity and eating disorders. *Psychiatr. Clin. North Am.* 2005 March;28(1):55-67, viii.

[30] Nasser JA, Gluck ME, Geliebter A. Impulsivity and test meal intake in obese binge eating women. *Appetite* 2004 December;43(3):303-7.

[31] Di M, V, Berrendero F, Bisogno T et al. Enhancement of anandamide formation in the limbic forebrain and reduction of endocannabinoid contents in the striatum of delta9-tetrahydrocannabinol-tolerant rats. *J. Neurochem.* 2000 April;74(4):1627-35.

[32] Di M, V, Matias I. Endocannabinoid control of food intake and energy balance. *Nat. Neurosci.* 2005 May;8(5):585-9.

[33] Sipe JC, Waalen J, Gerber A, Beutler E. Overweight and obesity associated with a missense polymorphism in fatty acid amide hydrolase (FAAH) *Int. J. Obes. Relat. Metab. Disord.* 2005 July;29(7):755-9.

[34] Hart CL. Increasing treatment options for cannabis dependence: A review of potential pharmacotherapies. *Drug Alcohol. Depend.* 2005 November 1;80(2):147-59.
[35] Huestis MA, Gorelick DA, Heishman SJ et al. Blockade of effects of smoked marijuana by the CB1-selective cannabinoid receptor antagonist SR141716. *Arch. Gen. Psychiatry* 2001 April;58(4):322-8.
[36] Huestis MA, Gorelick DA, Heishman SJ et al. Blockade of effects of smoked marijuana by the CB1-selective cannabinoid receptor antagonist SR141716. *Arch. Gen. Psychiatry* 2001 April;58(4):322-8.

INDEX

A

D

E

F

G

H

I

J

K

L

M

N

S

T

U

V

W

Y